An Action Guide to Job Hazards

W⬤rk & Health.

It's Your Life   Phillip L. Polakoff, M.D., M.P.H.

Press Associates, Inc.
Washington, D.C. 20005

PRESS ASSOCIATES, INC. is an independent news service which covers economic, political and social issues of importance to working people, particularly union families. PAI has been accredited to Congress for more than 30 years. Its news service goes to some 120 publications with a combined circulation of more than 12 million. In addition to the Work & Health column, PAI publishes Washington Window, an award-winning interpretive weekly column.

Copyright © 1984
Robert B. Cooney, Publisher
Press Associates, Inc.
806 15th Street NW, Suite 632
Washington, DC 20005
202/638-0444

Library of Congress Cataloging in Publication Data

Polakoff, Phillip L., 1945-
   Work and health.
   1. Industrial hygiene.   2. Occupational diseases—
Prevention.   I. Title.
RC967.P65   1984   613.6'2   84-61087
ISBN 0-918763-00-2 (pbk.)

Printed in the United States of America
Designed by Anne Masters
International Standard Book Number: 0-918763-00-2 (paper)

Dedicated to my mother,
Goldie B. Schwartz

Contents

3 Physical Agents: NOISE, LIGHT, HEAT, COLD, VISION, RADIATION & VIBRATIONS

4 Occupational Stress

Resources

Foreword

An overriding question facing all who are concerned with suffering, disease and death from occupational disease is where to focus one's efforts. There is so much to do. Shall we mount more research, to learn more about those agents, those circumstances, which cause disease? Should we help design laws and regulations to control these causes? Is priority to be given to on-site inspections to monitor existing regulations or is it best to concentrate on industrial hygiene engineering to assist industry in making the workplace safer?

All of these, and more, are important: union safety officers, epidemiologists, legislators, toxicologists, engineers, statisticians, industrial hygienists, experimental pathologists, administrators, occupational physicians, chemists, nurses, and others add to continuing and complex efforts to control occupational disease.

Dr. Polakoff has included these contributions in the chapters of his text. But he has gone beyond them, not only by their synthesis and interdigitation into a coherent whole, but with the entire perspective of what he has done. For he has taken the fertile past twenty years of progress in occupational studies and recast, molded and analyzed them *for use in the prevention of disease* — a noble aim, since occupational disease is primarily preventable disease. Not only "Here, this is what we know" but also, "This is how it can be used, these are the barriers, this is how they can be avoided. Above all, use this information, protect workers, save lives."

In this, he has followed the best tradition of occupational medicine, which acknowledges that while science is necessary, it is not sufficient. To best hold its goal of human good and its guiding spirit of compassion,[1] it must treasure its roots in the realities of the workplace. Ramazzini described how his remarkable, germinal treatise came to be written.

> *Scito, te genitum nigris Tabernis*
> *Non cultis Domibus Potentiorum*
> *Aut Aulis nitidis, ubi Archiatri*
> *Dictant Jura Coquis, sedentque nusquam.*
>
> *Si, qui te legerint, statim remittent*
> *Ad natalitias tuas Tabernas.*

You must know you were born in workshops
Not in elegant mansions for our betters
Not in glittering courts where chief physicians
Lay down laws for the cooks but sit down nowhere.

If they read you and straightway send you packing
Back to the workshops, remember — *you were born there.*

Bernardini Ramazzini, "The Author to His Book," in *De Morbis Artificum.*[2]

So it is with this volume. It was born amidst the day-to-day problems of workers and returns with what now can be done to alleviate them. In the best sense, this is what workers have the "right to know."

Irving J. Selikoff, M.D.
Mount Sinai School of Medicine
of the City University of New York

May 20, 1984

1 William Osler. The Evolution of Modern Medicine. Yale University Press, 1921, p. 6-7. "Medicine arose out of the primal sympathy of man with man." Osler quotes the medical historian Payne: "The basis of medicine is sympathy and the desire to help others, and whatever is done with this end must be called medicine."

2 Bernardini Ramazzini. Diseases of Workers, 1700. Translated by Wilmer Cave Wright, University of Chicago Press, 1940, from the Latin text of the Second Edition, 1713. Ramazzini's Address — ". . . an anxious father's warning" — is from the first edition, 1700.

Introduction

There is a struggle taking place every day in the workplaces of America, a struggle against accidents and disease. And the men and women in the mills and mines, in the offices and factories, and on construction projects are losing it. The death toll from on the job accidents is about the same as in the Vietnam war. Each year, approximately 5,000 workers are killed on the job. An additional 2 million are disabled. What is even worse is the toll from disease. Experts estimate that about 100,000 people a year die from occupational diseases which take time, but finally exact their price.

America has come a long way in recognizing these problems and the enormous human and economic toll involved. After years of legislative struggle, the public policy goal of a safe and healthful workplace was established with passage of the Occupational Safety and Health Act of 1970. Administration of the law focused on safety in the initial phase, with the government adopting industry codes wholesale. Later, advances in scientific and medical techniques and equipment laid the foundation for steady, if slow, progress against toxic substances, noise and other job disease-inducing agents.

The decade of the '70s also saw a boom in the occupation of industrial hygienist. Many unions and companies have employed these professionals to develop safety and health programs.

Unfortunately, the deregulation binge of recent years has halted or reversed some of the progress made during the first decade. Some industry groups and some powerful corporations took advantage of the pro-business political climate to momentarily halt the tide of change. So a rebuilding period lies ahead.

What has been most heartening has been the initiatives at the state and local levels. Alliances of union safety and health personnel and environmentalists and citizen groups have sprung up all over the nation.

The purpose of this book is to help shop stewards and managers and the men and women in the workplace become better informed about job hazards. With that knowledge, they can pursue resources in their union and company, in outside coalitions or in governmental agencies to make their workplaces safer and more healthful.

Phillip L. Polakoff

Acknowledgments

Jack Tucker made this book possible through his invaluable editorial guidance and assistance.

I would like to express my gratitude to all my colleagues at the Western Institute for Occupational/Environmental Sciences. Further appreciation is extended to various labor unions, government agencies (the National Cancer Institute, Occupational Safety and Health Administration, and National Institute for Occupational Safety and Health) and voluntary agencies which have supported my research and educational outreach activities over the last decade. I also would like to express appreciation to Margaret Seminario, AFL-CIO occupational health specialist, for her advice and assistance with resources in the labor movement.

The staff of Press Associates, Inc. played an important role in the preparation of this book. The articles which follow were syndicated to the labor press across the nation through PAI's weekly news service. PAI's staff edited the manuscript and researched the appendices. I thank Susan Zachem, Paula Campbell, Lynn Crawford, Donna Nielsen, Calvin G. Zon and Robert B. Cooney, Executive Editor of PAI.

I wish to thank my colleague and friend, Michael Smith, M.D., for his guidance and support. And, finally, my complete gratitude and love go to Nancy Pfund for her patience and understanding during this project.

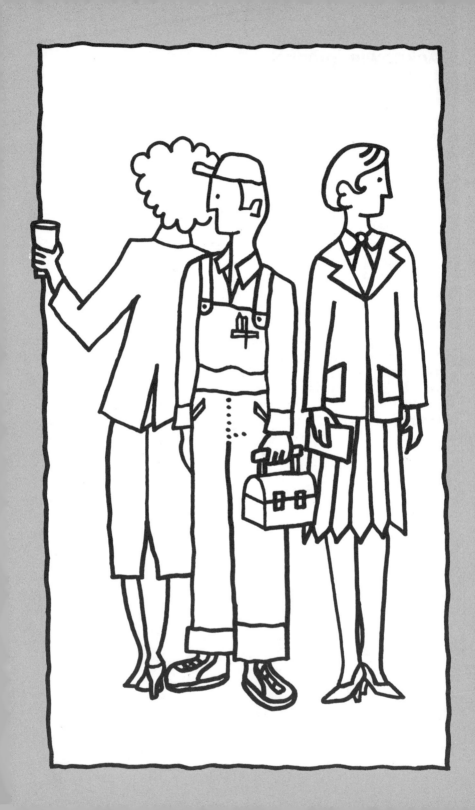

1 Job Safety & Health Issues

Old Problems, New Awareness

Contrary to what some people think, occupational diseases are not recent and unwanted offspring of 20th century technology. The growing awareness of job-related health hazards may be fairly new. So are the methods we use to detect them. But workers throughout history have been afflicted by the labors they performed.

Slaves toiling in the mines of ancient Greece and Rome were poisoned by such toxic metals as lead and mercury. Grinders, bending over their sandstone wheels in the 16th century, suffered from a respiratory illness called "grinders' disease" from inhaling silica dust.

But job hazards in the old days—even as today—were not limited to heavy industry. There were certain illnesses connected with occupations which we might refer to today as white collar.

Medieval scribes apparently suffered from lead poisoning as a result of shaping their quills with their tongues after dipping the quills into metallic ink solutions.

Sir Isaac Newton, the 17th century physicist who gave us the law of gravity, is said to have exhibited some strange behavior at one point in his life. It may have been a sign of mercury poisoning, rather than a scientist's quirk. Recent research tells us that Newton apparently spent his nights sleeping in his poorly ventilated laboratory where mercury compounds gave off toxic fumes.

Remember the antics of the "mad hatter" in "Alice in Wonderland"? His bizarre behavior may reflect as much fact as 19th century fiction. Workers in the hat industry were exposed to mercury vapors while treating fur to make felt. Some of them suffered such extensive brain damage that they actually appeared mad.

Although we now know that workers in the distant past suffered ill effects from their labors, even partial relief has been a long time coming. As far back as 1700, Bernardo Ramazzini, the first "occupational health specialist," suggested "cautions" that should be taken to safeguard workers in various trades. But nearly 300 years later, thousands of workers are still unprotected. Ramazzini also recommended that any doctor taking a case history inquire about the patient's occupation. But such obviously useful information is still not routinely recorded.

As early as 1914, life insurance companies in the United States denied policies to asbestos workers and uranium miners. Checking their mortality tables, insurance underwriters knew, perhaps more than anyone else, that these workers faced serious risk of early death from cancer and lung ailments. It is a sorry chapter in American industrial history that tells how most of these workers were not warned of the dangers by their employers.

Fortunately, things are changing. Scientists, physicians, workers and the general public now know more than ever before about occupational diseases. Unlike their forefathers, workers today have the legal right to protection against job hazards. They also have the right to compensation for diseases identified with particular industrial processes or trades.

Workers have a responsibility, too. They must become informed about how to use these rights and protections. However, before acting, workers must know what causes the occupational illness, who is at risk, and what self-protection is available. Unions have performed a great service in this respect.

A giant step forward on behalf of workers was taken by Congress with the passage of the Occupational Safety and Health Act of 1970. Under the law, employers have a "general duty" to provide a workplace free of hazards, and they must comply with standards issued by the Department of Labor's Occupational Safety and Health Administration (OSHA).

The Act also created the National Institute for Occupational Safety and Health (NIOSH) within what was then the Department of Health, Education and Welfare (now the Department of Health and Human Services). NIOSH conducts research on job hazards, and recommends new standards to OSHA.

Other government agencies charged with helping to safeguard workers' health include: the Mine Safety and Health Administration (MSHA), which oversees working conditions for mine and mill workers; the Nuclear Regulatory Commission (NRC), which sets safety standards for workers exposed to radioactive substances; the National Cancer Institute (NCI) which, along with NIOSH, gathers information about cancer hazards that may lead to the setting of new standards; and the Environmental Protection Agency (EPA), which has a mandate to control pollution in the areas of air, water, solid waste, noise, radiation and toxic substances.

The agencies and the workplace standards they develop and enforce are not perfect. But they represent an encouraging start toward dealing with an age-old problem.

The vital ingredient in making things work better is an informed rank and file that can spur government and industry to meet their legal responsibilities. After all, it's your health and life that are on the line.

A National Issue

How big is the problem of job-related disease?

According to the U.S. Department of Labor, there are more than 100,000 new cases of occupational disease every year. However, the department admits this figure includes only acute cases. Experts estimate many thousands more workers suffer from chronic or long-latent job disease, including job-related cancer.

There is another side to this problem that magnifies its severity. Occupational hazards pose threats to health that extend beyond the workplace itself. For example, workers sometimes expose their families to health risks by carrying toxic substances home on their clothing. Studies have shown that children of workers involved with lead dust have higher than normal levels of lead in their blood.

Even worse than lead poisoning is the threat to life from exposure to asbestos dust brought home from work. There are documented cases of death from cancer among women who washed their husbands' dusty clothes, and among children who played with their fathers after work.

The long reach of occupational diseases even extends to future generations. The National Institute for Occupational Safety and Health (NIOSH) has estimated that, of the 16 million working women of childbearing age, about 1 million are exposed to substances that could harm their unborn children.

And reproductive hazards are not limited to women. Substances such as lead and the pesticide DBCP can cause sterility and impotence in men. Both sexes are susceptible to genetic damage that can show up as birth defects in their children.

Wives of workers exposed to lead, vinyl chloride and anesthetic gases used in hospital operating rooms often have higher than average rates of miscarriages and birth defects among their children.

There is still another factor that further enlarges the problem of work and health. Factories that are hazardous places to work, because of the materials or processes used, also can pollute the entire community.

In addition to the ill effects on individuals caused by DBCP, the pesticide also has been found contaminating drinking water supplies in a number of communities. Likewise, the chemical kepone represented a hazard for the general population of a sizable area along the James River in Virginia as well as for the people who manufactured it.

In fairness, it must be said that health problems that originate outside the workplace can contribute to occupational illnesses and injuries. We bring to our jobs our own genetic makeup; our eating, drinking and smoking habits; our personal family problems; and our particular way of looking at and reacting to health and sickness.

One example of this interrelationship between occupational and non-occupational factors is the dramatic increase in the risk of lung cancer among asbestos workers who smoke.

Job-related disease or injury is a personal tragedy for workers and their families. But when we multiply these individual calamities by the nearly 2 million estimated victims, the problem widens to national scope.

Leading Job Diseases and Injuries

What are the 10 leading work-related diseases and injuries in the United States? Here they are, from a list compiled by the National Institute for Occupational Safety and Health (NIOSH):

1. Occupational lung diseases—asbestosis, byssinosis, silicosis, coal workers' pneumoconiosis, lung cancer, occupational asthma.

2. Musculoskeletal injuries—disorders of the back, trunk, upper extremity, neck, lower extremity; traumatically induced (that means caused by an injury) Raynaud's phenomenon. Sometimes this condition, affecting the fingers, may be brought on by the use of vibrating tools.

3. Occupational cancers (other than lung)—leukemia, mesothelioma, cancers of the nose, liver and bladder.

4. Amputations, fractures, eye loss, lacerations (cuts), and traumatic (injury) deaths.

5. Cardiovascular diseases—hypertension (high blood pressure), coronary artery diseases, acute myocardial infarction.

6. Disorders of reproduction—infertility, spontaneous abortion, teratogenesis (birth defects).

7. Neurotoxic disorders (nerve poisoning)—peripheral neuropathy (often characterized by weakness, muscle shrinkage, or numbness and tingling), toxic encephalitis (sometimes called "brain fever"), psychoses, extreme personality changes (related to toxic exposure).

8. Noise-induced loss of hearing.

9. Dermatologic (skin) conditions—dermatoses, burns (scaldings), chemical burns, contusions (abrasions).

10. Psychologic disorders—neuroses, personality disorders, alcoholism, drug dependency.

(NOTE: The various conditions listed under each category are only selected examples. They don't cover the whole field of these types of injuries or diseases.)

NIOSH used three measurements in compiling this list: how often the diseases or injuries occur, how severe they are, and how amenable the causes are to change for the better.

This list can serve several useful purposes, aside from satisfying the curiosity of American workers about the potential health and safety risks they may be facing on the job.

For one thing, the list should encourage a lot of thinking and debate among professionals (and that should include union leadership as well as medical people) about these major problems in the field of public health. For another thing, this list can help in setting national priorities for efforts to prevent health problems related to work.

The need for coming to grips with this problem is compelling. According to the latest available figures from the U.S. Department of Health and Human Services, nearly 5,000 workers die in job accidents each year. More than 2.5 million workers a year are disabled by injuries, 80,000 permanently. Approximately 21 million American workers are exposed to substances regulated by the Occupational Safety and Health Administration (OSHA).

Toxic effects have been reported for some 50,000 chemicals which are thought to appear in the workplace—more than 2,000 of which are suspected human cancer-causing agents in laboratory animal tests.

Every year, about one out of every nine workers in private industry will suffer an occupational injury, based on averages over the last few years. The costs of occupational accidents, both direct and indirect, are estimated at nearly $25 billion a year.

The 10 leading causes of illness and injury could well become the 10 most wanted criminals against American workers. They deserve to be tracked down and rooted out just as the lawbreakers who do violence against our persons and our property.

Is Your Job Making You Sick?

Finding out whether a health problem is job-related is a lot like a detective story:

- You have a crime—in this case, some harm to your body that's making you feel sick, or tired, or nervous, or whatever.
- You have a batch of clues (symptoms)—pain, swelling, rash, dizziness, nausea. The list could go on and on.

- You have the detective and his trusty sidekick—your doctor and you.
- And, like all good mysteries, there's a complication in the plot. In this instance, it's the fact that occupational diseases usually look and feel just like other diseases.

So how do we sift through the clues and nail the culprit as work-related instead of something you're doing off the job—smoking, drinking too much, overeating, not getting enough rest, or similar unwise personal habits?

An occupational history is a good way to start. If your doctor doesn't ask for one, suggest it. Here are some questions you should be pre-

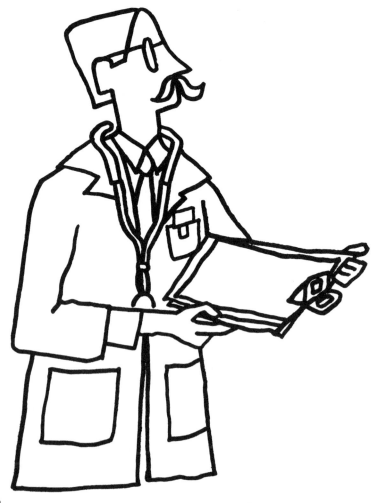

pared to answer. Not all of them will apply to every situation. This is just an outline to set you to thinking about your job and how it might be affecting your health.

What exactly is your job? Is it maintenance or production? What is the product? What materials (chemicals) are involved in the process? Do you have some idea of how the process works?

Is a list of plant chemicals you're working with, or exposed to, available? How about safety data sheets? Can you provide them?

Is your exposure airborne, something you can inhale? Can the suspected materials be absorbed through the skin? Can you ingest them, get them in your mouth from your hands when you eat or smoke?

Are excessive heat and noise a part of your work environment?

Have air samples (or other measurements) been taken? If so, when and by whom? Is the data available?

What, if any, ventilation is provided where you work? Can you describe it—type, location, etc.?

Are work rules and practices to control health hazards posted where you can see them? Are they being observed?

What personal protective equipment is provided? Is it used?

Is there a pattern to your disease or discomfort? Does it occur just during work and clear up on weekends or vacation? Does the problem show up more frequently among workers in a certain area of the plant, or among those only doing a certain job?

How many people are exposed? How often? For how long? How many shifts are there?

Besides your own immediate problem, are there any health complaints by your co-workers that you know about? How many complain? How often? Have they sought medical treatment? (A list of their names and the dates of their treatments would be useful.)

Are medical tests done regularly where you work? Are the records available?

Have you said anything about the problem to your union shop steward or safety and health rep? Was the information discussed with the company? Is the company doing anything about it?

The answers to such questions can be useful to your doctor as a medical detective on the trail of an occupational illness. If your health is suffering because of your job, or the conditions you have to work under, it is important to pinpoint this causal relationship:

- to protect your own health and the wellbeing of your family;
- to buttress any workers' compensation claims that may arise;
- to prod employers into complying with the health and safety laws that have been fought for and won in your behalf.

Accidents: Who's to Blame?

The so-called "accident-prone worker" is a scapegoat often trotted out to stall effective safety measures. But an accident in many cases is not the result of clumsiness or momentary lapse of attention. It could be the conclusion of a long string of contributing factors.

Dr. Stephen Zoloth and David Michaels, MPH, occupational health specialists at Montefiore Hospital in the Bronx, pinpointed such factors in a special safety issue of *Occupational Health Nurse* magazine. They included: heat, noise, lighting, toxins, improper training, inexperience, fatigue, shift, variability of tasks performed, speed of work, and the type of production incentives used.

One study cited by the two specialists, for example, showed that accidents increased 25 percent with every 5 degrees Fahrenheit rise or fall from an optimal temperature mediated by humidity, air-flow and acclimatization.

Instead of putting the blame on the victims, perhaps we should look more closely at the "accident-prone workplace."

These places where accidents are waiting to happen are not only in hot and heavy industries. Let's look at the health care industry itself. Surely, one might expect that scrubbed-down, starched-up environment should be free of risks for employees. Unfortunately, that's not the case.

Dr. Jeanne Stellman, writing in the same safety issue of *Occupational Health Nurse,* cited excessive accident rates among nurses and kitchen workers. A recent survey of one medical center, she says, found that nurses accounted for 60 percent of reported accidents, although they represented only 33 percent of the workforce. Kitchen workers, who comprised only 10 percent of the workforce, reported 19 percent of the accidents.

Dr. Stellman, who was editor of the special issue of the nurses' journal, is executive director of the Women's Occupational Health Resource Center (WOHRC), School of Public Health at Columbia University in New York. Among hazards she listed are needlestick wounds which can allow infections to invade the body, injuries from lifting, improper storage of chemicals in laboratories and inadequate staff training.

Hospitals also get a going over from Patricia Cayo Sexton, author of *The New Nightingales: Hospital Workers, Unions, and New Women's Issues* (New York: Enquiry Press, 1982). As one hospital aide, a member of the Service Employees International Union (SEIU), told the author: "In an eight-hour day, an aide lifts about 3,000 pounds. She gives maybe 20 baths in the morning and lifts more than a man in an auto assembly plant. That's why her back goes."

Sexton is a professor of sociology at New York University and a trade unionist. Her research, sponsored by the Coalition of Labor Union Women (CLUW), is based on interviews with national and local union leaders, management, and women workers in hospitals in California and Pennsylvania.

Here's another excerpt from her book on the subject of on-the-job health and safety from a hospital worker's viewpoint: "People get toxic reactions from the gas used in sterilizers. Administrators like to talk about all the protection gear they'll give the workers, but they never talk about changing the kind of gas used so workers won't need protection."

Running like a dark thread through these observations about job hazards in the health care industry—traditionally top-heavy with women workers—is stress. Job stress is not unique in this industry. It plays a major role in accidents and general health everywhere. Working under stress for short bursts may improve performance. But prolonged stress takes its toll in such complaints as headaches, insomnia, gastrointestinal disorders and many more.

Burdened with these uncomfortable, potentially harmful distractions, workers may have more accidents. But they are not necessarily "accident-prone." The workplace and work practices may be the culprits.

The Human Side of Job Diseases

Although precise figures are hard to come by, authorities estimate that every year 100,000 American workers die from illnesses linked to their jobs. Another 100,000 workers or more annually become newly ill by exposure to various occupational diseases. These are shocking statistics. Unfortunately, that's about all many of us know about this problem—the cold statistics.

Yet behind these impersonal numbers are real people, just like you. It may help to bring home this annual toll of occupational hazards if we look behind the statistics and flesh them out with human beings.

Here are just three cases picked at random from my patient file. The names have been disguised to protect the confidential nature of the doctor-patient relationship. Otherwise, the people and stories are real.

Todd N. is a 23-year-old male, a welder by trade, presently unemployed. He has no past history of diseases. He doesn't smoke, drink alcohol, or use drugs. Both parents are still living and in good health. His hobby is physical fitness.

On the face of it, Todd would appear to be a man in the prime of a healthy young manhood with no physical problems. But that's not the case. He is bothered by chest pains, shortness of breath, runny nose, coughing up mucus, throat irritation, anxiety and depression. These symptoms were experienced for several months.

The problem was traced to an incident one day at the place where Todd formerly was employed. Working in a fairly close space, and using no protective equipment, he welded some galvanized metal fixtures. Although a journeyman welder, this was his first experience with galvanized metal and he was not told of the health hazard.

Todd had come down with a bad case of heavy metal fume fever. Due to the intensity of the exposure, he probably also had toxic pneumonitis. The aftereffects were lingering longer than usual. No wonder he was anxious and depressed about his future!

Rosa F., 31, had no past history of serious illness when she went to work two years ago in an automotive firm. She had never smoked, didn't use drugs, drank socially on occasion.

She did general office work and was also responsible for some cleaning chores. The shop area of the firm was just outside the door of Rosa's office. Shop work included sandblasting, spray painting and metal grinding. She described the shop area as very dusty.

Two months after going to work, Rosa developed a persistent cough, later complicated by severe episodes of shortness of breath and wheezing. On two occasions, she had to go to the hospital. After six months on the job, she resigned because of the adverse health effects. She has not worked since.

The problem appears to be allergic rhinitis, allergic bronchitis and asthma—possibly due to inhaling substances at the workplace. Since there was no history of allergies, respiratory problems, asthma, food intolerances or other factors which might otherwise account for her condition, Rosa very likely is a casualty of the workplace.

Fred W., 42, has been a criminologist with a state law enforcement agency for 20 years. He is a nonsmoker, drinks moderately on occasion, and has no history of childhood or adult diseases. He drinks two or three cups of coffee a day, and has done so for many years.

Recently he learned that benzidine, a solution he worked with frequently in blood stain analysis, could cause bladder cancer. Disturbed by this information, he sought medical advice and an examination was made. It confirmed his fears. A bladder cancer was found and surgically removed. I believe Fred's bladder cancer was caused to a significant degree by his exposure to benzidine in his work as a criminologist.

These are just three brief glimpses into the human side of the occupational health hazard statistics. Similar life stories lie behind all those other workers whose jobs make them sick.

The Right to a Safe Workplace

You have the right, under law, to a safe and healthful workplace. Your protection is guaranteed under the Occupational Safety and Health Act—one of the most important gains achieved for all workers under the strong leadership of the trade union movement.

But your legal rights are only as good as your knowledge of how to use the law. OSHA can't do it all. You have to do your part, too.

Here are some steps for making sure that you get the protection you are entitled to on the job. These highlights are from a booklet, "Combating Hazards on the Job," published by the Food and Allied Service Trades Department, AFL-CIO.

1. *Recognize hazards and suggest solutions to your employer.* Probably the best way to do this is through your health and safety committee. Put everything in writing—the conditions and the suggestions— and make copies. Give the employer one copy and put the other in union files.

2. *If the company doesn't take action in a reasonable time, call for an OSHA inspection of the workplace.* This can be done by the worker or an authorized union representative. Even if you can't cite a specific OSHA violation, you can still call for an inspection under the General Duty Clause, or Section 5(a)(1), which covers, among other things, conditions that common sense tells you are dangerous.

Although the law protects you against discrimination by your employer for filing a complaint, many workers still are fearful of losing their jobs. If you feel this way, you might consider having the union file the complaint. Make sure an individual is designated as contact person for OSHA.

You do not have to sign the OSHA complaint or, if you call in, to leave your name. However, there are some advantages of having your

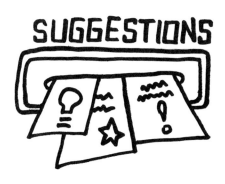

SUGGESTIONS

name connected with the proceedings. For instance, OSHA can contact you for clarification, or notify you if they decide not to make an inspection, or contact you after the inspection to explain what happened.

Workers are protected against discrimination by their employer for exercising their rights under the OSHA law. If you feel that you have been discriminated against, you have the right to file a complaint with the nearest OSHA office within 30 days. Remember that deadline; the 30-day limit cannot be extended.

If OSHA doesn't inspect immediately, or if your employer doesn't correct the hazard promptly, you can offer to perform other work until the hazard is corrected. If you are denied that option, your final alternative is refusal to do the work. But that is an extreme action and should be used as a last resort under the most serious circumstances. It may take months or even years to get your job back if you're fired. The law is hazy on this point.

3. *Participate in the health and safety inspection.* There are three parts to an OSHA inspection: The opening conference. The walk-around inspection. The closing conference. You have the right to participate in all three parts.

The AFL-CIO Food and Allied Service Trades Department suggests that you designate a representative to join you in the OSHA inspection. This individual probably should be on your health and safety committee.

Incidentally, since OSHA can't notify you or your employer in advance of the inspection time, it's a good idea to have a representative available on all shifts. The representative should be briefed on existing violations—where they are and when they occur. Your employer should be notified that you have a representative who will be taking part in the inspection.

A good walk-around representative is your assurance that the inspector gets your side of the situation and sees all areas you think are hazardous. The inspector should question affected workers about working conditions. You have the right to talk to the inspector in private, away from your employer. The more the inspector can learn about a job hazard, the better equipped he or she will be to determine if a violation exists. You cannot be penalized for talking with the inspector.

OSHA sometimes conducts routine inspections, in addition to those brought on by specific complaints. You have the same rights to participate in these routine checkups as you do for the complaint inspections.

Your right to a safe and healthful workplace was hard-won and is still being challenged. It is meant to be used whenever necessary—for your own sake as well as for the sake of your family and all who depend on your continued well-being.

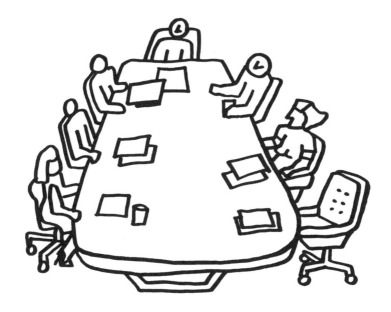

Workers' Compensation

"Worker compensation, they call it," said the husky middle-aged man in the blue windbreaker. "Making it up to me, I guess. But how can anybody compensate me for . . . " He paused and thrust forward his right arm that ended just above the wrist.

The woman, frail, in her 50s, has been a textile worker. Breathing with difficulty, she said: "It's better than nothing . . . but no amount of money can ever pay me back . . . for this . . . ." Her voice trailed off to a wheeze. Cotton dust had finally taken her off the job, but the mill would be a part of her life until death.

These are the victims of our industrial society. Their numbers are in the hundreds of thousands. This year, an estimated 100,000 workers will die from occupational diseases; more than 2 million will be injured in industrial accidents. About 1 in 10 of these injuries will leave the worker disabled.

As far back as 10 years ago, the U.S. Bureau of Labor Statistics revealed that one out of every eight workers suffered a "job caused" injury or illness. More recently, a study conducted by the University of Washington found that more than 50 percent of the workforce was suffering adverse health symptoms that could be attributed to hazardous substances or conditions in their work environment.

An estimated 8 million to 11 million workers have been, or still are, exposed to asbestos during the manufacture and installation of asbestos

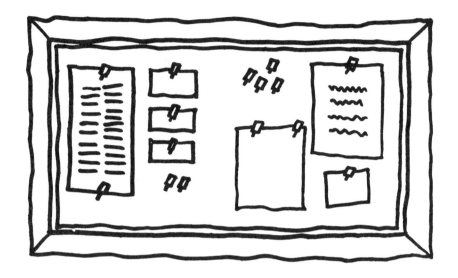

insulation and other asbestos products. Such exposure can lead to asbestosis, a form of fibrosis of the lungs, or to lung cancer. Even their families can be in peril, for the deadly fibers can be brought home from the plant on clothing. Sometimes the symptoms don't show up for years—20, 30, or even 40 years later.

At least 1 million workers hold jobs that expose them to free silica: miners of coal, iron, gold; stoneworkers; metal fabricators who use sand-forming casts; grinders and polishers of metal and stone; sand blasters. All of these workers risk developing silicosis, a lung disease that can be complicated by pulmonary tuberculosis.

For these victims of the industrial age, "compensation" is the wrong word. When a worker loses a hand or a foot or has his or her lungs destroyed, there is no way to "compensate" that worker or the family. No economic payment can ever make up for the loss of health—the inability to breathe or walk or just to perform normal functions of living. Money alone can't take the place of shattered family hopes in terms of food, housing, education, advancement and security.

Not that money is unimportant. There must be adequate financial help to tide workers and their families over the shoals of lowered income as a result of on-the-job injury or job-related illness. And the process of getting this help must be clear and simple.

It is not so simple now. How can a worker file a claim for an occupational illness—or a widow file for death benefits—when neither the worker nor his family really knows what hazardous substances he has been exposed to?

How can the victim get help when his personal physician, or the plant doctor (if there is one) doesn't know the trade-name products used in the plant? Or the multiple chemicals in these products? Or what their toxic effects are?

How can the worker, or the doctors, recognize an occupational illness or the toxic effects of the chemicals when the industry has not been required to pre-test the substances—and make the data available—before they are used?

What this boils down to is the need for more job-hazard information for workers. More toxicological data for professionals. A stricter testing system for industries to make sure of the safety of substances before they are introduced to the workplace and the market.

Yes, money is certainly important. But there are two other important needs:

1. Rehabilitation should become an integral and more effective part of the workers' compensation system. This will give disabled workers the chance to be productive again.

2. Occupational health and safety needs to come out of the dark and be better understood—not only for the sake of doctors and other health professionals, but for workers and employers as well. This will involve more and better testing, evaluating results, sharing the widest use of all the essential information, monitoring, etc.

This combination—adequate state and federal compensation laws, job retraining, and a better overall appreciation of occupational health and safety—finally will begin to provide true workers' compensation.

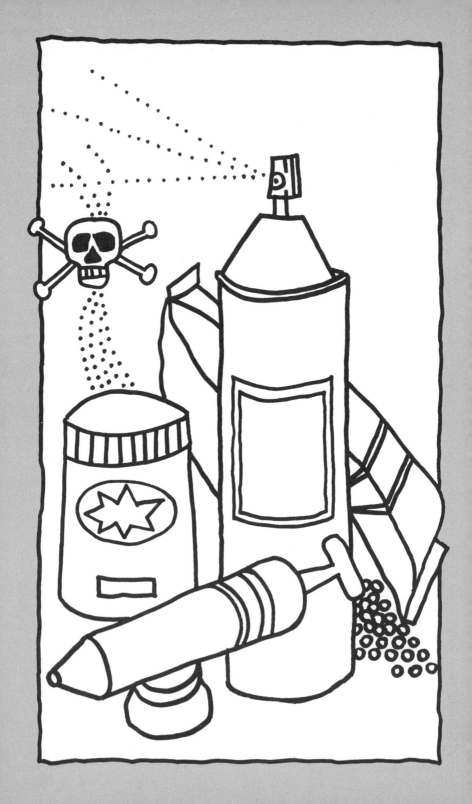

2 Chemicals in The Workplace

How Poisons Get into the Body

There are three ways for poisons to get into your body. You can breathe them. They can be absorbed through the skin. They can get in through the mouth and digestive tract.

The majority of poisons that affect your internal organs are breathed in. Substances like chlorine and ammonia can have an almost immediate irritating effect on the air passages and the lungs. Other substances may be absorbed from the lungs into the blood and cause damage to other organs.

Gases generally come to mind when we think about breathing something that's going to cause us harm. But there are many other substances, including heavy metals like lead, that also can be absorbed by breathing when they are in the form of fumes, vapors or dust. These fumes and vapors may be given off during various manufacturing processes when substances are heated or mixed. Welding is an example.

The skin has a natural barrier against injury by contact. This consists of a protective coating of oil and protein. But some chemicals can get through this thin barrier. Phenol or carbolic acid can penetrate the skin and you probably won't feel it. Other substances can burn their way through the skin and be absorbed into the bloodstream. From there they are carried throughout the body. The eyes and genitals, which have less protective skin covering, are particularly vulnerable to toxic chemicals. They can absorb up to 100 percent of the chemicals that touch them.

Ingestion, the third way poisons can get in, can happen in several ways. A worker whose hands are contaminated may carelessly touch his mouth. This can happen while smoking. Food may have been contaminated by handling or by being left exposed to toxic substances. Workers who handle extremely toxic substances such as lead or arsenic need to be especially careful about this hand-to-mouth contact.

What Is Toxic?

If a chemical or substance can cause harmful health effects, either long-term or short-term, in humans it is considered to be toxic. Whether you will suffer some harmful health effect after exposure to something that is toxic depends on any one of the following conditions, or a combination of them:

- What the stuff is made of, its chemical composition;
- The amount involved (a little of one substance might produce harmful effects ranging from mild to death, while a large amount of something else might be necessary to produce the same range of effects);
- Sensitivity of the individual (some people may get a severe reaction immediately from exposure that may have little effect on another person who is exposed to the same substance in the same way);
- Synergism (two or more substances acting together to produce an effect which neither would produce alone);
- Length of exposure (a one-time exposure of short duration may produce no harmful effect, but continued exposure even to small amounts each time, may produce harmful effects later).

Another important factor is how the substance is absorbed into the body or how the contact is made. This entry, or contact, can occur in a number of ways:

- You can inhale the substance because it is in the air you breathe.
- You can swallow it. This can happen if it's on your hands and contaminates food or whatever else you might touch and then put in your mouth. (This is an extra hazard for smokers.)
- The substance can get into your eyes.
- It can get on your skin, either directly from the source, or from contaminated clothing that touches the skin.
- Toxicants can also be transmitted by sexual contact.

Exposure can be either acute or chronic. *Acute exposure* is a single brief encounter with a toxic substance that may cause minor irritation. The effect generally wears off quickly after the exposure ends. Ammonia and chlorine, for instance, are two substances commonly used in industry which may cause immediate eye or respiratory irritation. These effects will disappear soon after the exposure ends.

Other substances are so toxic, on the other hand, that exposure to relatively small amounts can cause serious illness or death. In this group are such things as hydrogen sulfide, organophosphate pesticide, nickel carbonyl, and isocyanates.

Chronic exposure is repeated contact with a substance—even a small amount—over a period of time which can lead to serious health effects. Unfortunately, the ill effects of chronic exposure to a toxic substance may not show up for months or years. This delayed reaction may be due to the cumulative potential of the substance, piling up in the system over time, or because the effects are not completely reversed each time. These "time bombs" include asbestos, silica, lead and benzene. This is not a complete list, by any means, of substances that can cause long-term ill health effects. In fact, according to industrial hygienists, any substance—ANY substance—a person is exposed to at high levels can become toxic.

Employers have a legal responsibility to find out what substances in their workplaces may be unsafe or potentially harmful. The law also requires employers to inform their workers of any potential chemical hazards and to make sure workers are trained and equipped to work safely with these substances. Workers and union representatives also should insist on their "right to know" what substances they are working with and how they can protect themselves.

Common Toxic Hazards

Listed here are some common substances found in industrial plants. Following the name and descriptions are (1) common uses, and (2) possible health effects.

ASBESTOS (fibers of various sizes, textures and colors): *Uses:* Thermal and electrical insulation; filler for plastics and cement. *Effects:* Causes asbestosis, cancer of the lungs and digestive tract, and mesothelioma.

CADMIUM DUST/FUMES (soft silver-white metal). *Uses:* Electroplating, some silver solders, cadmium-silver batteries, protective metal coating, certain insecticides. *Effects:* Severe lung irritant, especially the fume; kidney damage, metal fume fever.

CARBON MONOXIDE (odorless, colorless, tasteless gas). By-product of incomplete combustion of gasoline, wood, etc. *Effects:* Headache, nausea, dizziness, weakness; at high concentrations can cause coma and death.

COAL TAR PITCH VOLATILES (volatile matter emitted when coal tar or coal tar pitch is heated). Occurs during pitch melting operations. *Effects:* Cancer of lungs, kidneys, skin; bronchitis, dermatitis.

EPOXY RESINS (liquid). *Uses:* Molding compounds, surface coatings, adhesives, laminating or reinforcing plastics. *Effects:* Dermatitis, lung irritation, nausea; may cause lung or kidney damage.

FORMALDEHYDE (pungent, irritating gas). *Uses:* Manufacture of leather, rubber, woods and metals (no-bake resins in foundries). *Effects:*

Skin, eye and respiratory irritation and inflammation; may cause cancer and genetic damage.

IRON OXIDE (red-brown fume with a metallic taste). *Uses:* Welding, grinding; often found in iron foundries. *Effects:* Pneumoconiosis (siderosis); gray iron lung disease.

LEAD, METALLIC LEAD, LEAD OXIDE (solid, heavy pliable metal; gray fume when heated). *Uses:* Storage batteries, paint, ink, ceramics, ammunition, brass/bronze foundries, some welding and soldering operations. *Effects:* Weakness, insomnia, weight loss, constipation, stomach discomfort, decreased appetite; in severe cases, kidney damage, sterility, birth defects.

METHYLENE CHLORIDE (colorless liquid with ether-like odor). *Uses:* Solvent in paint and varnish removers, insecticides, fire extinguishers. *Effects:* Fatigue, weakness, drowsiness, light-headedness, nausea, numbness of limbs, eye and skin irritation.

OZONE (blue gas with pungent odor associated with electrical sparks). Present around arc welding and electrical equipment. *Effects:* Irritation and dryness of the throat, headache, dizziness, burning sensation in the eyes, bronchial asthma, swelling of the lung tissue.

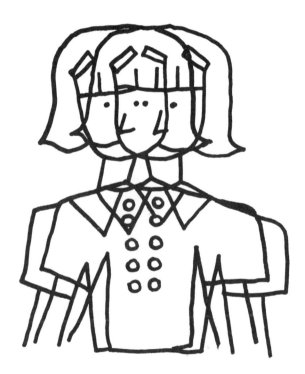

SILICA (colorless crystals). *Uses:* Manufacture of glass, porcelain and pottery; metal casting, sand blasting, refractory grinding and scouring compounds. *Effects:* Silicosis, a progressive, disabling and sometimes fatal lung disease, characterized by shortness of breath, wheezing, coughing and increased susceptibility to tuberculosis.

TOLUENE (colorless liquid with aromatic odor). *Uses:* Component of gasoline, solvent for paints, coatings and common cleaning agents. *Effects:* Weakness, fatigue, confusion, insomnia, dermatitis; may sometimes engender a feeling of euphoria.

XYLENE (colorless liquid with aromatic odor). *Uses:* Common solvent; a raw material used in manufacture of certain chemical compounds. *Effects:* Eye and skin irritation; dizziness, drowsiness, lack of coordination; can also cause skin conditions.

This is just a brief sample of some common substances found in the workplace. There are many, many more. Do not use the list of possible health effects for self-diagnosis. But do not ignore frequent headaches, colds and coughs, dizzy spells or skin and eye irritations. Check with your doctor.

Smoking, Toxics and Worker Health

Smoking is the single most important preventable cause of disease and death. Yet millions of people keep right on puffing, undermining their health and shortening their lives. Why?

One reason, suggested by research studies, is that people who are generally aware that smoking is harmful don't relate the risks directly to themselves. Knowing that "smoking is dangerous" is not the same thing as believing that "smoking will hurt ME." Another reason, these studies indicate, is that smokers may be vaguely aware that smoking isn't good for them but they don't know exactly what the bad effects are, or how they show up. Or they grossly underestimate the ill effects.

So, if you're still smoking, or thinking about taking it up, here are some specifics you might want to take to heart—literally:

Statistically, you're going to die younger than someone who has never smoked; younger than those who quit.

If you smoke, the chances of coronary heart disease killing you is about one and a half to two times higher than for nonsmokers, according to the U.S. Department of Health and Human Services. The rate is three times higher if you're a man 45 to 54 years old and are a heavy smoker—a pack a day or more.

Men who smoke die of lung cancer at a rate 10 times higher than nonsmokers. Men who smoke more than two packs a day have a death rate 15 to 20 times higher. Lung cancer is the leading cause of cancer death among men.

And the lung cancer risk is growing for women smokers. Their death rate is now five times greater than among nonsmoking women. If present trends continue, it soon will be the leading cause of cancer deaths among women.

Cigarette smoking during pregnancy is associated with retarded fetal growth, and increased risk for spontaneous abortion and prenatal death. Slight impairment of growth and development during early childhood has also been noted among the children of mothers who smoked during their pregnancy.

Chances of developing chronic bronchitis or emphysema skyrocket for smokers. The death rate for those who smoke less than a pack a day is four times higher than for nonsmokers. If you smoke more than a pack a day, your chances zoom up to seven times higher. If you cough a lot to bring up phlegm and are short of breath when you exert yourself, you are showing some of the typical symptoms of chronic bronchitis. Check with your doctor.

With emphysema, the tiny air sacs in the lungs lose their elasticity, rupture and are destroyed. The lungs can no longer expand and contract easily for breathing. Emphysema also puts an added burden on the heart which must work harder to pump oxygen-starved blood through the damaged lungs.

Workers exposed to toxic materials in the workplace run an even graver risk from smoking than the general population. In some cases, smoking has a multiplying effect when it interacts with other toxic substances. This can result in more severe health damage than from either the occupational exposure or smoking alone.

 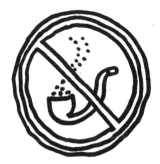

Asbestos provides one of the most dramatic examples of this "synergistic" effect. Studies show that smokers who are exposed to asbestos have eight times the risk of lung cancer as all other smokers, and 92 times the risk of nonsmokers who are not exposed to asbestos.

Fortunately, present evidence suggests that people who quit smoking cigarettes can improve life expectancy, although not back to that of the nonsmoker. Ten years after quitting cigarette smoking, the death rate for lung cancer and other smoking-related causes of death approaches that of nonsmokers. The choice is clear. Sticking to it takes guts.

Job Dusts—Mineral, Organic, Chemical

Dusts form wherever solids are broken down to smaller particles. Nature has been kicking up dust this way since the beginning of time, using the forces of sun, wind, water and microorganisms to decompose plant and animal matter into soil; and wearing down boulders to make sandbars and beaches. Man makes dusts by speeding up this natural process, using such mechanical means as drilling, blasting, crushing, sawing, grinding and so on to reduce raw materials to more manageable and useful sizes.

However they get into the air we breathe, dusts can be hazardous to our lungs. To guard against this long-standing and universal hazard, our breathing apparatus has developed a remarkably efficient system of housecleaning.

The nose filters out many of the larger particles. When finer particles breeze past this first line of defense, they can be trapped in other air passages lined with a thin layer of watery mucus. These passages also are lined with cells containing hairlike extensions, called cilia, which sway slowly and constantly in an upward motion to move the mucus into the windpipe. There, we swallow it subconsciously or spit it out.

The coughing and sneezing mechanisms also are triggered to help us get rid of the irritants. Deeper in the lungs are cells that surround and attempt to digest the dusts and other airborne lung hazards, or to herd them into various drainage channels.

This elaborate cleansing system works well for most people most of the time, although its efficiency may vary from person to person. Trouble comes when the system gets overloaded, as in a very dusty workplace, or when other burdens are added—notably cigarette smoke and general air pollution. Cigarette smoking also hastens the progress of lung diseases that already may have taken hold.

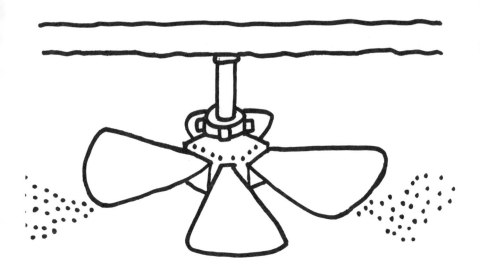

Depending on their origins, dusts are classified as mineral, organic or chemical.

Mineral dusts come from rocks, stones and ores found in the earth's crust. Any workers involved with mining, crushing, loading, hauling and refining of these materials can be exposed to their dusts. Smelter workers and those employed in other refining processes—potters, brick and tile makers, stonecutters, metal workers—all can be exposed to the same mineral dust hazard.

Organic dusts come from living things such as plants, animals and microorganisms. Dust is given off when these materials are harvested, transported, stored or processed—milked, chopped, spun, sawed, pulverized and so on. Animal and poultry handlers can be exposed to hair, dander and feathers, all potential dust sources. Tiny seeds or spores produced by fungi are another troublesome source of organic lung hazard.

Chemical dusts are generally powdery forms of synthetic chemicals, such as bleaching powders, pesticides, dyes or catalysts used in various manufacturing processes.

Most mineral dusts are not dissolved or broken down by lung tissue. They tend to accumulate in the body and cause irritation which can lead to chronic bronchitis, emphysema, fibrosis (a stiffening of the lung tissue) and cancer.

Organic dusts, on the other hand, generally are dissolved in the lung fluids or broken down by bodily processes. They don't usually accumulate in the lungs. Instead, they may set off a hypersensitivity reaction. Coarse organic dusts may provoke occupational asthma. Finer particles can penetrate to the alveoli, the tiny air sacs at the very end of the lung system. Certain wood dusts also have been linked to nasal cancer.

Chemical dusts can produce a variety of lung damage, depending on the various properties of the chemicals involved. Some are irritants, such as fluoride; others are caustic—sodium hydroxide, potassium hydroxide, chloride of lime (bleaching powder)—and can inflict chemical burns when inhaled. So many new dry chemicals have been introduced into the workplace over the last decade that their long-range health effects have not yet had time to be evaluated. Some may cause cancer, but we may not know it for years because of the long latency involved.

There are three principal ways to reduce hazardous dust:

1. Changing machinery, ingredients and work practices to eliminate or reduce the amount of dust generated, contain it better or separate it from people;
2. Ventilating the area to reduce dust concentration and prevent build-up;
3. Providing personal protective equipment as a back-up measure when the first two preferred methods don't do the whole job.

Asbestos Is Everybody's Problem

Asbestos used to be thought of as a health hazard only for asbestos workers. Not any more. Millions of people on and off the job (including school children) face the potential risk of breathing the tiny fibers that can cause a number of serious diseases. Why? Two reasons:

1. The large amount of asbestos mined and processed in the U.S.—about 800,000 tons a year.
2. The wide range of uses asbestos is put to—some 3,000 products, two-thirds of them used in the construction industry. These products include reinforced asbestos cement sheets and pipes, pipe insulation, roofing felt and shingles, floor tiles, patching and taping compounds, brake linings, clutch facings, insulating paper and protective clothing.

Asbestos becomes a health hazard when fibers are set free in the air where they can be breathed. This usually happens when the asbestos material can be crumbled in the hands. "Friable" is the technical term. Common examples are old insulation, or ceilings sprayed with asbestos for fireproofing, soundproofing, decoration and so on.

Most sprayed asbestos was banned in 1978 by the Environmental Protection Agency (EPA). But some spray jobs done before that time are still in place and may cause problems. The EPA says, for instance, that between 5 and 15 percent of the nation's public schools contain some asbestos materials. It's also found in many other buildings and private homes.

Asbestos floor tile, on the other hand, isn't "friable." The fibers are firmly bound or sealed into the tile. The trouble comes when this sealed type of asbestos is cut, ground or sanded.

Asbestos dust can cause asbestosis, a lung disease, and cancer of the lung and other parts of the body. In asbestosis, the fibers lodge in the lungs, irritating them and causing inflammation. As the inflammation heals, it leaves scar tissue that eventually can stop the air in the lungs from getting into the bloodstream. This can lead to slow suffocation or heart failure, but most deaths are due to secondary respiratory infections like pneumonia and bronchitis. Infections most often can be treated if the person gets prompt medical attention.

The first sign of lung cancer may be a persistent cough, or a change in the cough habit. Chest pain, a sort of aggravating ache, is the second most common symptom. Blood-stained sputum coughed up from the lungs is sometimes another early sign.

Not all the inhaled fibers stay in the lungs. Some are rejected and can move up the throat where they may be swallowed. This can lead to cancer of the esophagus, stomach, intestines and rectum. Once asbestos gets into the body, it stays indefinitely.

Lung cancer and cancer of the esophagus can be treated by surgery, drugs, radiation, or a combination tailored to each individual. Cancer of the large intestine or rectum is curable, in many cases, by surgery, especially if detected early. Tests are available to improve the chances of early detection.

Mesothelioma is a rare form of cancer of the membranes that line the chest and abdomen. It is hardly ever found in people who have not been exposed to asbestos. Most often, it is fatal.

Nobody knows why yet, but asbestos exposure may make one person sick and not harm somebody else working side by side under the same conditions. But we do know that the risk of getting lung cancer rises as the length of exposure increases. This risk goes up dramatically among smokers. Asbestos workers who smoke are about eight times as likely to get lung cancer as those who don't smoke.

It's up to employers to protect workers from asbestos. That's a worker's lawful right. There are a number of ways to do this:

Engineering controls. This means isolation and/or enclosure of operations, exhaust ventilation, and dust collection, among other things.
Product substitution. Using a safer material, like fiberglass. But fiber-

glass itself can cause skin and eye irritations, sometimes severe. More study is needed.

Handling procedures. Whenever practicable, all asbestos should be handled wet.

Housekeeping. All external surfaces must be kept free of fiber buildup.

Respirators. A backup safety device. Workers who can't function normally when wearing a respirator cannot be given a job where respirators are required. When respirators are used, workers should be shifted around so they are not exposed all the time.

Clothing. The employer must provide special clothing, change rooms, clothes lockers and laundering. (CAUTION: Don't take work clothes home to be washed.)

Monitoring. Employers must measure the amount of asbestos fibers in the workplace air regularly, and let workers see the records.

Medical examinations. Workers must be given medical exams, including chest X rays and breathing tests, when they are hired, once a year while they are working, and at the time they leave the company.

Asbestos In Auto and Truck Repair

Nearly every worker faces possible exposure to asbestos because the material is used in so many ways in so many different places. Resistant to both acid and heat, this strong and durable mineral is used in a variety of products and processes—from insulation and floor tile to brake linings and clutch facings.

Let's consider just one group—auto and truck repair workers, particularly those who handle clutch and brake jobs. Much of the following information is taken from a booklet produced by Machinists Local 1101, San Jose, Calif., in cooperation with the staff of the Western Institute for Occupational/Environmental Sciences, Berkeley, Calif.

If you work in an auto or truck repair shop, here are some of the more common ways you can be exposed to asbestos dust: removing wheels with air tools; removing wheel covers, hub caps and beauty rims; balancing wheels; cleaning wheels; rotating tires; and changing tires. Any brake or clutch work also involves the possibility of exposure.

People who don't actually do these jobs, but who work in the same garage or shop, also can be exposed. Asbestos can break down into tiny, sharp fibers so small you can see them only with an electron microscope. Because of their small size, these fibers can remain airborne for long lengths of time and cling to clothing and hair, exposing people some distance from your worksite. You can even take this deadly dust home with you, risking exposure of your family.

Here are some general ways to prevent asbestos exposure:

- Wear an approved asbestos dust mask while working on a job where you might be exposed.
- Use the vacuum or wet method to keep the dust down. Never blow asbestos dust with an air hose!
- Isolate jobs on which exposure is possible; for example, do brake work in specific areas only.
- Avoid eating in areas where there is asbestos dust.
- Make sure to change your clothes after work and wash up before you leave.

For tire work, spray the wheels with water, using a spray bottle, before removing the wheels with an air gun. This will reduce the amount of dust blowing into your face and the air. The same precautions about wetting down the area applies to clutch work and brake jobs. Clutch facings and brake linings or shoes contain asbestos. The fibers are present in the dust that collects on clutch plates and brake drums.

Never scrape asbestos dust—dry or wet—onto the floor; it can become airborne. Instead, scrape the wet or dry dust into a container. Empty the container into a plastic bag and seal it tightly. Label the bag "ASBESTOS." Remember, somebody else may be emptying it and unknowingly get exposed. Wear an approved asbestos dust mask while doing this clean-up.

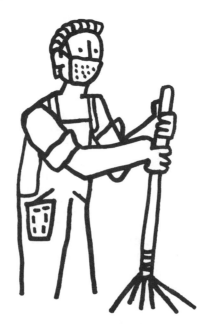

There are some pros and cons for these safety techniques. But the odds greatly favor playing it safe in light of the serious health hazards involved with asbestos exposure.

Blowing the dust away may seem like a fast and efficient method. But this is extremely hazardous, exposing not only the worker, but other people. Using the wet method of dust control involves the cost of containers or bags and maybe a slight bit of extra time. If solvent instead of water is used to wet down the area, there is the possible added risk of breathing the solvent mist or vapors. But this is a safe and effective method, well worth the extra cost and time. Also, disposing of the container is easy.

Fitting a vacuum device to the brake drum is sometimes difficult and time consuming. Cleaning and storage are extra chores. But with a proper fit, the vacuum method is safe and effective. This method is recommended by the State of California and some unions.

A final reminder: there is no known "safe" level of exposure to asbestos. There is no definite amount of time that can be called "safe" for a worker to be exposed. The safest known exposure is none at all.

The Battle against Silicosis

To say that the subject of silicosis is "breathtaking" may border on shockingly bad taste. But that's what silicosis does to its victims—literally takes their breath away. And if that's shocking, so is the pitiful amount of data gathered in 30 years about how much silicosis still exists among foundry workers, miners and people who are exposed to silica dust in ceramic, glass and granite work.

The International Molders and Allied Workers Union is now taking on this job. The union's Health and Safety Department is collecting and analyzing inspection records of the U.S. Occupational Safety and Health Administration, workers' compensation claims and results of medical screening tests. The goal is to get a clearer idea of the extent of silicosis in foundries represented by the union. This is a commendable effort which, hopefully, can help to point the way toward eliminating the threat of this deadly lung disease caused by inhaling silica dust.

Silicosis develops in the air sac region of the lungs when very fine silica particles slip past the respiratory filter system. If you can imagine a tree growing upside down from your windpipe (representing the tree trunk), the air sacs would correspond to tiny buds at the ends of the farthest-out branches. This is the area of the lungs where oxygen in the air you inhale is exchanged for the carbon dioxide in the blood.

41

When silica dust reaches the air sacs, they react with a get-tough defense in an effort to repel the foreign invasion. Unfortunately, this can lead to formation of scar tissue. The thick fibers can limit the ability of the lungs to stretch. This, in turn, means that less air can be drawn in. Sometimes the scar tissue can cover so much of the walls of the air sacs that there isn't enough surface area for good oxygen exchange. The result is an obstruction of breathing, similar to emphysema.

Silicosis progresses slowly, but relentlessly. There is no known medical treatment. It may not show up for 10 or 20 years or longer after the first exposure. However, it has been known to develop after 3 to 5 years of exposure to heavy concentrations of dust. And there are rare cases of acute reaction in as little as 1 to 3 years after exposure to extreme concentrations, such as in closed spaces.

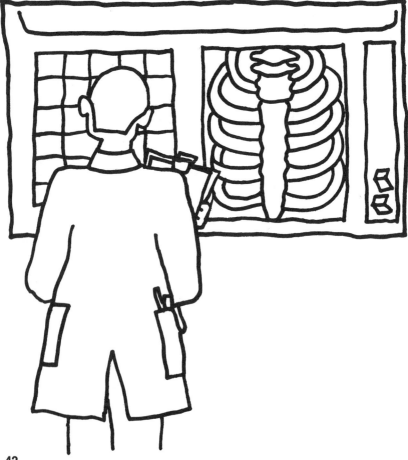

Frequent dry coughing, shortness of breath, wheezing and increased tiredness are warning signs of silicosis in its early stages. These symptoms get worse as the disease progresses. Death generally results from respiratory failure, heart failure (from the increased strain of trying to breathe), pneumonia or other complications.

Doctors rely on three main tools to diagnose silicosis:

1. *Chest X rays.* These can show the scar tissue mentioned earlier. It is important that the X rays be examined and interpreted by a medical person experienced in looking for silicosis. Exposed workers should have a chest X ray at least every 2 or 3 years to detect the disease in its early stage.

2. *An occupational history.* Silicosis is just one of a family of diseases caused by inhaling dust particles. There is also asbestosis from inhaling asbestos fibers, and black lung caused by coal dust. The job history can help to pin down the culprit that's causing the problem.

3. *A lung functioning test.* These tests should be conducted every year by a qualified pulmonary technician to track any changes in the workers' ability to breathe.

The most effective way to reduce the risk of silicosis is to prevent exposure in the first place. This could mean substituting a less toxic non-silica material wherever possible—olivine or zircon sand, for example, in molds and cores. Metallic shot, slag products or grit could be used in sandblasting operations.

Some risk can be "engineered-out" with the use of exhaust hoods and ventilated booths, or by remote control of sand slingers. Good housekeeping—vacuuming and wet sweeping—can remove settled dust before it is kicked back into the air.

Although useful, respirators should be considered a last resort after substitution, engineering and housekeeping.

Silicosis needs the kind of aroused public awareness and action that has been given to asbestosis, black lung and brown lung among textile workers. The more this devastating disease is brought out into the open and its risks reduced, the easier will foundry workers, miners and their families breathe.

Understanding Brown Lung Disease

Brown lung, or byssinosis, is one of a family of diseases caused by inhaling tiny particles of dust—in this case, dust from cotton, flax or hemp.

The disease is a particular hazard for textile mill workers. It is most likely to develop among susceptible workers in the carding, picking and opening rooms of the mills where dust concentrations tend to be high. It can also affect workers in other areas such as the winding and weaving rooms if there is enough cotton (or flax or hemp) dust in the air.

Byssinosis can develop any time in a textile mill worker's life, although it usually begins after a short exposure. The first reaction is like an asthma attack: tight chest, shortness of breath, "air hunger" and a dry cough. There is a curious pattern in the way the disease develops. Unlike what you might expect, it doesn't build up during the work period, say, Monday through Friday, with the worst coming at the end of the week. Instead, brown lung sufferers usually get an attack when they return to the mill after a few days off—a weekend or vacation. Because of this pattern, the disease has sometimes been called "Monday fever." The symptoms may even clear up as the week goes on and not reappear until the next Monday.

Later, however, as the disease continues its course, the symptoms may last through Tuesday and Wednesday and eventually the entire week. Once brown lung has reached this stage, it may persist even when there is no dust exposure, even after retirement.

The labored breathing associated with brown lung is caused by the narrowing of the medium and small tubes in the lungs, and an excess build-up of mucus in the tubes. The air has a hard time moving out of the tubes and makes a wheezing sound.

This difficulty of air to get out results in back pressure on the lung's tiny air sacs which can rupture their delicate walls, leading to emphysema. The resultant strain on the right side of the heart has been fatal. Repeated exposure has led to chronic inflammation of the air tubes, or chronic bronchitis.

Since byssinosis affects the way the lungs work, rather than their appearance—as in the case of the scarring associated with asbestosis—chest X rays may appear normal. The chronic bronchitis or emphysema of a brown lung sufferer may look like the same conditions resulting from cigarette smoking or long-term exposure to other industrial substances like nitrogen dioxide and chlorine.

Brown lung diagnosis, therefore, generally is based on a combination of the symptoms, occupational history, and measurement of breathing capacity during exposure.

Byssinosis, like all lung diseases, is difficult to treat. The first step is to reduce the amount of dust and other irritants breathed into the lungs. Smoking should be cut out completely. Added to cotton dust exposure, smoking increases the likelihood that byssinosis will be serious, and raises the risk of other chronic lung complications.

Some people with byssinosis can be helped by bronchodilators. As the name suggests, these can dilate, or open up, the narrowed air passages. When chest infections occur, they may be treated with drugs prescribed by a physician.

As further treatment, the doctor may advise a change in the job, after giving the patient a thorough physical examination and studying the working conditions. Sometimes, a change to another job in the same mill may be helpful, if the new area is free from the offending dust that caused the problem in the first place.

There are federal standards for acceptable levels of cotton dust, as well as for work practices in the cotton processing industries. But until the problem has been brought fully under control, workers exposed to cotton dust should be aware of the lung hazards they are facing and have regular medical checkups. .

Gases: Useful but Dangerous

Gases—the air-like form of fluids that can expand indefinitely—are among the most valuable and most dangerous substances in the workplace.

They provide fuel—butane, propane, acetylene, for example. They are used as ingredients in chemical reactions. These include oxygen, hydrogen, ammonia, chlorine, fluorine, bromine, phosgene and countless others. They even provide jobs in the sizable industries that manufacture gases for industrial and domestic consumption. Gases are essential for such specialized purposes as anesthetics and life-support systems in medicine.

But there is a darker side to this picture. Wherever gases are manufactured, handled, transported or used, there is a potential risk to both health and life.

Gas-producing chemical reactions can be either natural or man-made. Nature produces gases during the fermentation process. Fresh silage ferminating in a silo, for example, can result in highly toxic nitrogen oxides, posing a threat to farm workers and their families. Even entering a poorly ventilated empty silo has sometimes proved fatal. The decay of organic matter in sanitary landfills and sewage treatment plants may produce both hydrogen sulfide—the rotten egg smell—and methane gases.

The interaction of solar ultraviolet radiation and oxygen produces ozone, a toxic and irritating gas, in the upper atmosphere. There are reports that it has proved troublesome for some people in high-flying air-craft. Ozone is also produced by the action of sunlight on photochemical smog from automobile emissions. Certain welding operations also give off ozone.

Various gases are produced in industries where high-heat processes are used. The American Lung Association, writing about occupational lung diseases, points out several such dangers:

> Welding and brazing can, in badly ventilated areas, allow a build-up of dangerous gases like ozone and nitrogen oxides. If these operations are conducted anywhere near chlorinated hydrocarbons, such as degreasing agents, phosgene—a highly dangerous gas—may be produced. Smelting, oven-drying, and furnace work are other potential sources of hazardous gases.

Fire fighters encounter hazardous gases such as phosgene and nitrogen oxide from burning synthetic materials used in many modern buildings. Hydrogen cyanide, carbon monoxide and carbon dioxide are also occupational hazards for fire fighters.

Phosgene and nitrogen oxide are among the gases that do not have an immediate irritating effect on the upper respiratory tract. The reason for this is that they are not readily soluble in water and don't quickly reach the tissue beneath the watery lining of the upper air passages. But this only increases the danger. Since there is no early warning, these gases have a chance to go deeper into the lungs, slowly attack the tissue, and do extensive damage before the first symptoms occur. This may be many hours after the exposure.

There are other gases that have just the opposite properties. They dissolve readily in the watery mucus lining the nose and throat, go to work on the underlying tissue, and the victim knows almost immediately that he or she is in trouble. These gases include ammonia, chlorine, bromine and sulphur dioxide.

Gases do their harm in various ways. Some that are fairly inert, like nitrogen and methane, can suffocate a person simply by displacing oxygen in the air. Some are poisonous to various body systems: hydrogen sulfide attacks the central nervous system; carbon monoxide prevents the blood from picking up oxygen. Even oxygen itself can be toxic at elevated pressures—as in diving.

Isolation of potentially dangerous operations, substitution of less hazardous substances, adequate ventilation: These are all possibilities that managements should explore to reduce the risks to workers' health and lives.

Where gas masks are required, make sure you have a good fit, that the canister is in good operating condition, and of the right type for the particular hazard you may be exposed to.

Carbon Monoxide—Invisible Killer

Carbon monoxide is one of the most dangerous and widespread industrial hazards. The main source of this invisible, odorless gas is the incomplete burning of anything that contains carbon. This includes gasoline, natural gas, oil, propane, coal and wood.

Every year, some 2,000 persons are killed outright by carbon monoxide. At least 10,000 more workers suffer from exposure high enough to cause serious health effects. Millions of others experience milder effects. These figures are not precise because there is good reason to believe that a large number of cases of carbon monoxide poisoning, both fatal and non-fatal, go unreported or incorrectly diagnosed. The symptoms are fairly general, especially at relatively low levels, and might suggest other causes. Carbon monoxide also aggravates other disease conditions, particularly heart trouble and respiratory difficulties.

The most frequent source of carbon monoxide in the workplace is usually the internal combustion engine, although coke ovens, blast furnaces and forges also produce the gas. Among those obviously at risk are operators of lift trucks, front-end loaders and diesel engines, as well as those working nearby. When such equipment is operated in an enclosed area, the risk is particularly dangerous. Such areas would include garages, filling station repair shops, warehouses, dock areas, the holds of ships during loading and unloading, vehicular tunnels, toll collection stations and so on.

Carbon monoxide poisons its victims by displacing oxygen in the blood. Oxygen from the lungs normally is carried through the body by the blood's hemoglobin. But when carbon monoxide is inhaled, the hemoglobin grabs the poison first, passing over the available oxygen. This explains how workers can die within a few minutes because of large amounts of carbon monoxide in the air, even though there is also plenty of oxygen available.

Tests have shown that carbon monoxide combines with hemoglobin 210 times as fast as oxygen does. Without oxygen moving through the blood stream, the victim suffocates. At lower levels of concentration, carbon monoxide takes over part of the oxygen-carrying function of the blood. The effects vary with individuals, but the most common complaints are headaches, nausea, drowsiness, tightness across the chest, tiredness and inattention. As exposure increases, the worker may become uncoordinated, confused and weak. Continued exposure can lead to convulsions, coma and even death.

High doses of carbon monoxide—even if the victim recovers—may cause permanent damage to body tissues that require a lot of oxygen, particularly the brain and the heart.

47

Besides being a health hazard, carbon monoxide is a safety hazard as well because of some of the effects just mentioned. A worker whose coordination is affected, or who becomes drowsy on the job, is a likely candidate for an accident and a risk to others. There are two basic approaches to eliminating this hazard to health and safety:
1. Get rid of the source.
2. Get rid of the gas itself.

Some businesses—warehouses, for example—have eliminated the source by switching to battery-operated fork lifts which give off no exhaust. This is a good solution, particularly in the winter when doors and windows generally are closed and the risks from gasoline-burning equipment are particularly high.

Another idea that has proved effective is to enclose dangerous operations and install blowers or fans to carry away the gas. The exhaust system should be installed in the ceiling or high above the source of the carbon monoxide. The gas is slightly lighter than air and, when it comes from a tailpipe, is usually hot and has a tendency to rise.

Many tunnel attendants and toll collectors are provided with glass-enclosed booths and an independent fresh air supply. Newer tunnels have built-in exhaust fan systems that turn on automatically when the level of carbon monoxide reaches dangerous levels. Portable blowers, properly placed, can dissipate carbon monoxide in other situations, such as on shipboard where longshore workers labor between the decks.

A word of caution: Just because you can't see or smell the exhaust from an internal combustion engine doesn't mean that carbon monoxide isn't present. Remember, this gas is invisible and odorless. The blue or white plumes you see are other gases or water vapor. The killer strikes without warning.

Two Irritant Gases

Sulphur dioxide and nitrogen dioxide are just two of a number of lung-irritating gases that workers can be exposed to in a variety of jobs. Where would you most likely find these gases? What do they smell like? What are some of the effects of breathing them? How can you best protect yourself? Here are some of the answers.

Sulphur dioxide is produced by chemical plants; petroleum refineries; the smelting of copper, lead and zinc ores; even the burning of trash. Industrial uses range from manufacturing ice to bleaching beet sugar to preserving fruit.

Despite such "sweet" uses, however, sulphur dioxide smells terrible. In fact, the strong, suffocating odor of the colorless gas will often drive people out of the area before acutely toxic concentrations are inhaled. On the other hand, some people get hardened to the smell. This tolerance increases the risk of deep lung irritation because the individuals can be exposed to higher concentrations for long periods of time.

Sulphur dioxide is readily soluble in water, and is especially irritating to moist tissue. This combination of traits explains why sulphur dioxide is so potentially harmful to the surface of mucous membranes of the throat and lungs. Contact with sulphur dioxide may bring on a dry throat, a cough or a burning sensation in the upper respiratory tract. If the exposure continues, you may notice fatigue, loss of the sense of smell, shortness of breath and increased mucus production.

People with a history of lung ailments and cardiovascular diseases, as well as the elderly and children, should be especially on guard against exposure to high sulphur dioxide levels.

Management must supply proper ventilation and, in many cases, supplied-air respirators. When the sulphur dioxide is in liquid form, protective clothing (including goggles and gloves) should be worn. This equipment should be washed at least twice a week. You should shower after each work shift.

Nitrogen dioxide can enter the atmosphere from a variety of sources—as a by-product of natural gas combustion, in industrial processes using nitric acid, and from motor vehicle emissions.

On-the-job exposure is just as varied as the sources of the gas. It is used in the making of rocket fuels, dyes, fertilizers, chemicals and pharmaceuticals. Other uses are in jewelry making, lithography, gas and electric arc welding, food bleaching and electroplating. Even the farmer filling his silo may run a risk.

Unlike the foul-smelling sulphur dioxide, nitrogen dioxide has a sweetish odor. Nitrogen dioxide is one of a very few colored gases. Its reddish-brown hue is what gives smog its characteristic color.

Nitrogen dioxide is not very soluble in water, but it does take place. And the slower rate of solubility means that the delayed formation of nitrous and nitric acids penetrates deeply into the lungs and slowly attacks the tissues. Because it doesn't smell too bad and acts so slowly, nitrogen dioxide may do extensive damage before the first symptoms occur many hours after exposure.

Proper respiratory and eye protection is a necessity if you work in confined spaces where nitrogen dioxide may accumulate. A supplied-air respirator with a full facepiece or chemical goggles should be worn. Enclosed areas should be properly ventilated before workers enter. In particularly hazardous situations, it is recommended that an observer be stationed outside the area with appropriate respiratory equipment to provide aid if needed.

You should have regular medical checkups and tell your doctor about your occupational exposure. With this information, he or she can look for signs of skin, eye, lung and heart diseases. (NOTE: Cigarette smoke contains a high concentration of nitrogen dioxide. This form of self-pollution is a major contributor to respiratory disease.)

Ammonia Can Be Harmful

Of all the irritant gases a worker's nose might get a whiff of on the job, probably none is more instantly recognized than ammonia. Even if the refrigerator in the lunchroom conks out, people don't ask: "What's that funny smell?" They say: "I smell ammonia."

There's no need to describe the pungent odor in terms of something else—like rotten eggs for hydrogen sulfide, or putrid fruit for phosgene. The word "ammonia" alone is enough to wrinkle your nose.

Workers in many industries are familiar with the smell. Ammonia is used in making fertilizers, explosives, dyes and plastics. Quantities of ammonia are used in such industries as refrigeration, petroleum refining, chemicals, pharmaceuticals and leather tanning.

As an occupational hazard, ammonia is peculiar. It is not a poison. It is not an additive—that is, it doesn't build up in the body with repeated exposure. Lung injury is rare—for the simple reason that most workers, unless they are trapped and escape is impossible, get out of the area before acutely toxic concentrations are inhaled.

But this doesn't mean that there are no risks with ammonia. Because the gas is so readily soluble in water, it is intensely irritating to moist surfaces. That's why your mucous membranes, eyes and skin react so quickly to the sharp, stinging sensation. Your breathing passages and throat are the first to feel the suffocating clutch. High concentrations can cause uncontrolled coughing, difficulty in breathing, and eventually suffocation.

Ammonia gas can produce headaches, excessive saliva, burning of the throat, perspiration, nausea, vomiting and pain below the sternum (breastbone). In liquid form, ammonia can cause first- and second-degree burns if spilled on your skin. Contact with your eyes can cause blindness.

But one of the biggest dangers of ammonia—not often thought about by many workers—is the possibility of fire. In high concentrations, ammonia gas will burn. Unless good housekeeping practices are followed, the gas can combine with oil and other combustibles and multiply the danger of fire.

Strange as it may seem, considering ammonia's overpowering pungency, some people can become conditioned to it. On the other hand, others may develop a hypersensitivity. Either way, for these people the hazards of ammonia are increased.

A person who is tolerant of high concentrations runs a greater risk of deep lung irritation, possibly without knowing it until the damage is done. At the same time, hypersensitized persons may experience an asthma-like attack following a milder exposure. Higher concentrations could be fatal.

The hazards associated with gaseous ammonia can best be controlled by ventilation. Exposure limits have been set at 50 parts per mil-

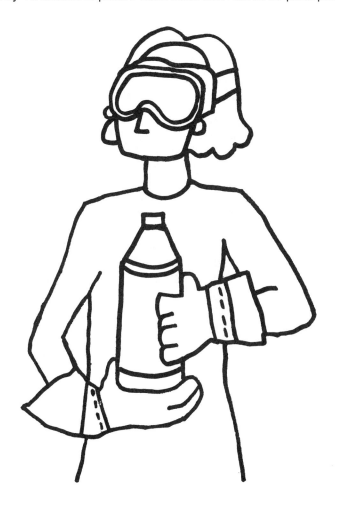

lion of air for an eight-hour period. If the concentration goes above that average, full-face gas masks or supplied-air respirators should be provided. By all means, wear them!

When liquid ammonia is involved, goggles or face shields and protective clothing (including gloves, aprons and boots) are required. If you should get a splash of ammonia in your eyes, immediately flood your eyes with large quantities of clear water for at least 15 minutes. Then get medical help.

There's one other personal protection measure that's entirely up to you. Cigarette smoking is dangerous to your health, no matter what your job is, or where you work. Because smoking increases the risk of lung disease, people who work with irritant gases—like ammonia and all the others—should seriously consider quitting. As the American Lung Association says: "It's a matter of life and breath."

TDI—More than an Irritant

When the Space Age blasted into public awareness some 25 years ago, one of the many exotic chemicals that came into widespread use in the wake of the new technology was one called TDI, short for toluene diisocyanate (also known as tolyene diisocyanate). Today, just as spacecraft launchings have become almost commonplace, TDI has become a familiar ingredient (and hazard) for workers making polyurethane plastics, various foams, coatings, adhesives, fibers and rubbers.

An estimated 40,000 American workers may be exposed to TDI on the job, according to the National Institute for Occupational Safety and Health (NIOSH). Among them are organic chemical synthesizers, aircraft workers, boat builders, mine tunnel coaters, ship welders, spray painters and wire coating workers.

Others who may have to deal with TDI hazards at one time or another, according to NIOSH, are abrasion-resistant rubber makers, adhesive workers, insulation workers, lacquer workers, plastic foam makers, plasticizer workers, polyurethane sprayers and polyurethane workers, textile processors and upholstery makers.

TDI is primarily an irritant, rather than a life-threatening chemical. It irritates all living tissue it touches, especially the mucous membranes of the eyes and the respiratory tract.

Contact with liquid TDI makes the skin redden and swell. Inhaling too much TDI vapor can cause nausea, vomiting and abdominal pains, as well as breathing problems. Splashed in the eyes, TDI will cause severe irritation and tears.

Fortunately, most of these ill effects appear to be temporary and the victims of TDI overdoses should suffer no lasting problems provided they receive treatment and are not exposed repeatedly to high levels.

However, a small number of people—probably about two out of 100—are not so lucky. These workers can become "sensitized" to TDI vapors. When that happens, scientists believe that the TDI chemically alters protein in the lung tissue of those individuals, causing the body to attack the altered protein. The result can be a severe allergic reaction, leading to a full-blown asthmatic attack. Victims wheeze, have great difficulty in breathing and experience a feeling of tightness in the chest.

The sensitizing process rarely takes place on a first exposure to TDI. The usual pattern of sensitization follows weeks or even years of repeated exposure. But once sensitized, a worker can experience a reaction after even a very low level of TDI exposure. In fact, there is no safe concentration for workers sensitized to TDI, to the best of present knowledge.

Since TDI is the product of chemical reactions that take place in a closed system, it is not too hard to control exposure to the vapors at the point of manufacture provided the system doesn't break down or an accident happen during maintenance.

The real problems of exposure come in the many industrial applications. Here are some suggested solutions:

- Enclose or hood such fixed-location operations as a rigid foam-mixing machine and provide downdraft ventilation. Ventilation face velocity of 200 feet per minute should be adequate for vapor control.
- Within 10 feet of spraying operations, workers should wear positive-pressure, air-supplied hoods; impervious gloves, tightly buttoned coveralls, and foot protection. Unprotected workers—those without gas masks—should not come within 50 feet of outside spraying operations.
- Wear cup-type chemical goggles if there is any chance of TDI splashing into the eyes. Protective clothing and rubber shoes, or rubber coverings over safety shoes, should be worn to guard against all skin contact with liquid TDI.
- Clean up spills promptly with a mixture of water, ammonia, and isopropyl alcohol.
- Sample the air periodically. You can't smell TDI in the air until the concentration is well above the permissible level.
- Don't eat or smoke in TDI areas, and don't wear your work clothes home.

Lead Poisoning

Lead poisoning is one of the oldest known—and sneakiest—occupational diseases. Old, because lead has been used in manufacturing for so long in so many different ways. Sneaky, because lead can damage your body, and the health of your family (especially children), in so many different disguises.

You can get lead poisoning from fumes, dust, paint and other compounds containing lead. That means the hazard can be lurking wherever there's heat, sanding or grinding, spraying, or the handling of lead-containing materials—chemical mixing, ceramics and pottery.

And the risks don't stop at the source. You can contaminate your house if you bring home lead-contaminated work clothing and shoes. Studies have shown that the children of lead workers had higher concentrations of lead in their blood than the children of other workers in the same neighborhood. Children are much more susceptible to the effects of lead than are adults.

In a commendable educational effort, the United Auto Workers has compiled a helpful worker's guide to lead exposure and the right of workers to receive protection from this ancient menace. The UAW points out how the earliest symptoms of lead poisoning can come on gradually and may be often overlooked. It's a long list of common complaints, including headaches, fatigue, irritability, nervousness, sleeplessness, pains in joints, aching muscles, poor appetite, stomach pains, constipation and high blood pressure.

"Gee," you might say. "That takes in everybody I know, sometime or other." And you'd be right, of course. But if you're a lead worker and have any of those symptoms persistently, see your doctor.

There are other signs that are more clearly warning signals to lead workers: severe stomach pains, weakness, a blue line on the gums, wrist drop (a type of paralysis), tremors, convulsions and kidney failure. Some health problems are so sneaky you probably can't feel them—anemia, nerve damage, sterility. Whatever the problem, obvious or hidden and only suspected, be sure your doctor knows you work with lead.

Lead enters the body primarily by inhalation. It can also be ingested, that is by mouth, if you eat food or smoke when your hands are contaminated with lead particles. Lead usually can't penetrate the skin, except in special chemical forms such as tetraethyl lead in gasoline.

Once in the body, lead zeroes in on four main targets—the blood, the kidneys, the nervous system and the reproductive system:

- Lead poisons the hemoglobin manufacturing system of the red blood cells. (Hemoglobin is the chemical inside of the red blood cells that carry oxygen from the lungs to all parts of the body.) When the body tissues are starved for oxygen, anemia results. This causes fatigue. Severe anemia can lead to heart failure.

- The kidneys take a beating because these are the organs which cleanse lead from the blood.
- Lead acts on the nervous system by slowing nerve impulses. This can interfere with coordination, and cause changes in personality and loss of memory.
- High levels of lead exposure are reported to cause sterility and a higher rate of spontaneous abortion and stillbirths in women and defective sperm and sterility in men.

Lead can be stored in the bones and released years after a worker has stopped being exposed. This delayed effect of lead poisoning is often due to stress, poor nutrition or alcoholism.

Companies have a responsibility under the law to control lead hazards through engineering techniques and good work practices. It is not enough to provide respirators or, even worse, transfer workers in and out of high lead jobs in a kind of human "yo-yo" control method.

All workers exposed to lead should be given regular blood tests. How often depends on the exposure level. Complete medical examinations are required for workers with levels above 40 micrograms of lead per cubic meter of air. Ask for the results of your tests and the company doctor's report so you can give them to your doctor. If there's anything you don't understand, ask questions. It's not only your right; you owe it to yourself—and to your family.

Welding Fumes

Eddie McB. was feeling on top of the world when he donned his welder's gear that Monday morning after a long weekend and got ready to work on the boiler. The feeling didn't last long. About an hour later, he said to a buddy, "I feel like I'm coming down with the flu."

Eddie had all the flu symptoms. He felt chilled and feverish at the same time, his head was aching, he was thirsty, and generally pooped. But he had the wrong name for what was ailing him. As any old-timer could have told him, Eddie was suffering from metal fume fever, an illness to which welders are particularly susceptible.

Metal fume fever seems to hit workers most often after a few days off. The reason for this is that your body may develop defenses against the fumes during the regular workweek. This defense mechanism tends to relax, just as you do, during a weekend or layoff for a few days.

When you start back on the job, the body has to gear up again to protect you. That's why the symptoms rarely last more than a day or so. Apparently there are no lasting effects from a small "dose."

But don't let the usually short duration of metal fume fever, or its apparent lack of lasting health effects, lead you to underestimate the hazard of welding fumes in general. Different types of welding operations give off different fumes which can produce dangerous and lasting effects. Shake them all together, and welders face a witch's brew of dangerous substances.

The fumes of brass are the most common cause of metal fume fever. The more zinc there is in the brass, the worse the fumes. Aluminum, antimony, cadmium, copper, magnesium, manganese, nickel, silver, tin and zinc also have been known to cause the disease.

Toxic fumes are given off during welding when the base metal and electrode are heated. Here are a few welding materials and their fumes' toxic properties, symptoms and health effects:

Galvanized steel. This metal can produce zinc oxide fumes and cause chills, nausea, throat dryness, exhaustion and fever. These are the symptoms of metal fume fever mentioned in the case of Eddie McB.

Stainless steel. Chromates and fluorides can be given off by this metal. Symptoms include irritation of skin, eyes, nose and throat; nose bleed and general weakness. These fumes have the long-term potential of causing nose ulcers, lung cancer, and bone disease.

Mild steel. Iron oxide and oxides of nitrogen can be produced by this material. These can cause eye, nose and throat irritation and possibly damage the lungs. Iron oxide is suspected by some investigators to be a factor in lung and liver cancer.

Aluminum. Ozone and phosgene are among the fumes given off in aluminum welding. Both are irritating to the air passages and can lead to a condition commonly called "water in the lungs." Ozone may cause chest pains. Phosgene exposure may result in chills, dizziness and thirst among other symptoms.

There are two main ways to protect workers from welding fumes. Ventilation is the best way to eliminate the hazards. If ventilation is not practical—where the work space is cramped, for example—respirators must be worn.

Mechanical ventilation of 2,000 cubic feet per minute for each welder is a suggested minimum of good air. This amount should be increased when welding is done with electrodes larger than 3/16 of an inch (1/8 inch with flux cored electrodes). Mechanical ventilation is generally required when space is less than 10,000 cubic feet per worker, or in a confined space, or where structural barriers restrict ventilation.

As for respirators, always wear them when toxic substances are present, even though there is no immediate risk to life or health. The type should be an air line respirator, a hose mask, or a respirator with an appropriate canister/filter. Canisters are painted in different colors to indicate which contaminant they are effective against. Be sure you use the right color canister for a particular welding fume hazard. If you're in doubt, ask your shop steward.

No matter what type of respirator you use, to be effective it should be approved by NIOSH (National Institute for Occupational Safety and Health) or other competent authority. Look for the approved label on the respirator.

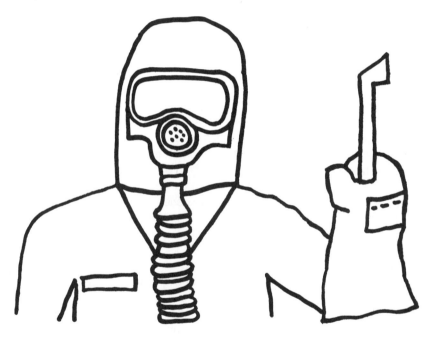

Handling Mercury

Mercury is one of the oldest metals known to man. It first got the name "quick silver"—probably because it is liquid at room temperature—around 350 B.C. Even the ancient Romans recognized it as a poison.

Today, nobody can escape mercury. Traces of the metal are everywhere—in the air, water and food. We aren't sure what is a "normal" level of mercury in the human body. But scientists are certain of one thing: at high levels, mercury is dangerous and can cause a wide range of physical and mental problems. Workers exposed to mercury on the job, or who come in contact with contaminated materials, run the risk of adding to the body burden of mercury that everybody carries.

A few years ago, the National Institute for Occupational Safety and Health (NIOSH) estimated that some 150,000 people may be exposed to mercury at work. These workers include mercury miners and refiners; embalmers; boilermakers; producers and users of disinfectants, insecticides, fungicides and bactericides; investment casting makers; electronic device makers; electroplating workers; and measuring instrument makers. Also people who make and load explosives and munitions; dentists; chemical and medical laboratory workers; paper, paint, ink and dye makers; amalgam makers; gold and silver extractors; leather and fur processors; taxidermists; wood preservative workers; photographers, and fingerprint detectors. Because it vaporizes at temperatures as low as 10 degrees Fahrenheit, the colorless, odorless vapor could be present anywhere mercury is used.

Spilled mercury creates a lot of potential problems. The silvery white liquid usually breaks up into tiny beads that can lodge in cracks, mix with dust, and penetrate such porous materials as wood, tile, iron pipe, and firebrick. Mercury also can cling to clothing (especially knit fabrics) and to the soles of shoes. This means that a worker can take the health hazard home and endanger family members.

Breathing the vapor is the most common cause of mercury poisoning, although mercury also can enter the body through the skin and the digestive system. Acute poisoning can be caused by short exposures to high levels of mercury. The victim may experience tightness and pain in the chest, difficulty in breathing, inflammation of the mouth and gums, fever and headache.

Far more common than such an acute episode, however, is chronic poisoning caused by long-term exposure to lower levels of mercury. Although the body is constantly getting rid of some mercury—in the urine, feces, and perspiration—steady exposure can cause a slow build-up if you add a little more daily than you get rid of.

Besides inflammation of the mouth and gums, victims of chronic mercury poisoning often show such symptoms as weakness, an increase of saliva, loss of appetite and weight, and trouble with digestion and the kidneys. When the central nervous system is involved, the effects often show up as tremor, or shaking, especially in the hands.

Some victims of chronic mercury poisoning show marked personality changes—such as irritability, outbursts of temper, excitability, shyness and indecision. Scientists also have found that long-term exposure, even to very low levels of mercury, can reduce a worker's reaction time and interfere with the ability to perform delicate tasks.

Limiting exposure to mercury is the best way to prevent the damages it can cause to workers' health. This can be done in several ways:

- By ventilation of areas where mercury or mercury compounds are handled;
- By enclosing and isolating mercury processes;
- By regularly monitoring the work environment and the status of workers' health;
- By good housekeeping to control the accumulation of mercury in the workplace;
- By good personal hygiene to prevent contamination of clothing, food and personal articles.

Cutting Fluids—Triple Threat

If the roster of occupational health hazards was an imaginary football team, a top choice for a triple-threat backfield position would include cutting fluids. These fluids, used to cool and lubricate cutting edges and metal workpieces in machining operations, can come at you in three different ways: by penetrating the skin and reaching underlying tissue and the bloodstream; by passing through the nose and throat in the form of oily mist which can become stuck in the lungs; and by entering the digestive system through the mouth when food, chewing gum or tobacco are contaminated by the cutting fluids.

There are four basic types of cutting fluids:

1. *Insoluble oils* are usually mineral oils, but many contain animal or vegetable fats and oils. Some also may contain additives, such as sulfur or chlorine, to make them work better under high cutting pressure and heat.
2. *Soluble oils* are oil-in-water emulsions. They also may contain additives which prevent rusting, foaming or formation of bacteria, make a smoother mixture or one better able to stand up under pressure.
3. *Synthetic fluids* are water-based, with organic and inorganic chemicals added for lubrication. They also may contain anti-rust, anti-foam, anti-bacteria and pressure-resistant agents.
4. *Semisynthetic fluids* are synthetic fluids with oil added.

Whatever the type and whatever path they take to get inside you, cutting fluids can harm the body in several ways. Studies show that workers exposed to insoluble cutting oils have a greater chance of developing cancer of the skin, respiratory system and digestive tract than non-exposed persons.

Many base oils and additives are irritating to the skin and can cause skin allergies. Symptoms include rashes, itching and pustules. Cutting oils also can plug up the skin's hair follicles, leading to formation of pimples, blackheads and acne.

The same additives that cause skin allergies also can affect the respiratory tract. Symptoms include shortness of breath, wheezing and coughing. Continued exposure may lead to pneumonia. Inhalation of cutting oils also may cause scarring of the lungs. This condition can make breathing difficult and interfere with the lungs' job of providing the body with the oxygen it needs to function normally.

To protect workers, the Occupational Safety and Health Administration (OSHA) has adopted a permissible exposure limit (PEL) for oil mist. This OSHA standard limits the exposure of workers to no more than 5 milligrams of oil mist per cubic meter of air, averaged over the workday. However, this standard has not been revised to include the data on the cancer-causing ability of oil mist. This means that exposure to even less concentration than the present permissible limit could still cause adverse health effects, especially over a long period of time.

If you suspect that you are being exposed to more oil mist than is good for you, look for these signs: haze around lights, poor visibility in the shop, stinging of eyes and nose, difficulty in breathing.

Accurate measurements of oil mist concentrations require taking a personal air sample and analyzing it using a technique known as fluorescence spectroscopy. In the sampling procedure, exposed workers wear portable pumps on their belts. These devices draw air through a membrane attached to the workers' shirts and positioned within 6 inches of the nose and mouth. These samples from the breathing zone are taken during the entire workshift. At the end of the shift, the filter is removed and sent to the lab, along with a sample of the cutting fluid being used.

There are several steps that can be taken to reduce the hazards of exposure. It may be possible to cut down on the amount of a known cancer-causing agent in the fluid, or to find a less toxic substitute which will still do the job as well. If mists are being generated by the machining operation, the work area can be enclosed and provided with an exhaust system. Overlapping, drip-proof splash guards can be installed around the operation to prevent workers from being splattered with oil. Preventive maintenance can reveal leaking lines and seals that should be replaced.

Workers can help themselves by using protective clothing when they cannot avoid contact with the oils. Respirators should be worn to guard against mist inhalation when ventilation is inadequate. Remember, respirators must fit you to be effective. If you are given a respirator to wear, ask to have it fitted before you use it. Only use respirators that have been approved by the National Institute for Occupational Safety and Health (NIOSH) and/or the Mine Safety and Health Administration (MSHA). The NIOSH/MSHA approved respirators will have the letters TC along with a number stamped on them.

Industrial Solvents

If somebody told you So-and-So was "two-faced," you'd probably be on your guard, never knowing his pat on the back was just a way of finding a soft spot to stick it to you. Right?

Industrial solvents, unless you're careful, can be like that. They come in handy for many operations, dissolving materials like oils, greases and resins. They are also mixed in with a variety of products, including paints, varnishes, lacquers, adhesives, plastics, textiles, waxes and polishes. But industrial solvents also can be "two-faced." Turn your back on them, in a manner of speaking, and they, too, can "stick it to you" and harm your health.

You should be especially on guard against breathing the vapors from organic solvents. This is the main way they can get into your body. Certain solvents also can be absorbed through the unbroken skin. The most common result of skin contact is dermatitis—inflammation of the skin.

By far the most serious damage, however, comes through inhalation. Overexposure can damage the lungs, blood, liver, kidneys and the nervous system. The stomach and intestines—the whole digestive tract—are vulnerable to highly toxic or irritating solvents. These include benzene, carbon tetrachloride, carbon disulfide, and formaldehyde.

Sometimes with certain solvents, if the exposure was not too concentrated or didn't last too long, the ill effects may go away after awhile with no apparent permanent damage. After too many whiffs, you might feel drowsy or befuddled and uncoordinated. But even these passing effects can increase the risk of accidents.

Don't take any of these warning signs lightly. Carbon tetrachloride—which can cause drowsiness, dizziness, headaches and fatigue—may affect the normal functioning of the brain. Severe exposure can cause unconsciousness. Extensive or continued overexposure, in some cases, has resulted in liver and kidney damage.

Carbon disulfide may cause damage to the motor nerves that control the body's voluntary movements after chronic exposure. Benzene is a notorious enemy of the blood-forming tissue of the bone marrow. Also, there's strong evidence suggesting a link between benzene exposure and leukemia.

Formaldehyde vapors are extremely irritating to the mucous membranes of the nose and throat. High exposure can lead to inflammation and edema, that is, a swelling of the passageways to the lungs. Formaldehyde is also believed to be carcinogenic (cancer-causing).

There are a number of ways of controlling exposure to hazardous solvents. As always, the best place to start is at the source of the hazard. This may mean changing the way a job is done. Continuous or automatic filling of vats, for example, might be used in place of manual batch-filling. Switching to a solvent that is less toxic and that doesn't evaporate so quickly might be another possibility. Local exhaust ventilation is an effective way of keeping vapors away from the worker's breathing zone.

Next in order come protective clothing, respirators and good personal hygiene. Gloves and aprons should be worn to prevent skin contact. If there is a possibility that solvents could be splashed into the eyes, then safety glasses, goggles or face shields should be worn. Count on respirators only for short-time, intermittent or emergency use. Respirators should not be used as a regular means of protection against solvent vapors. Exhaust ventilation is usually required.

Wash splashes off the skin as soon as possible. Change clothing that has become soaked with solvents. And if you smoke, think seriously about knocking it off, because cigarette smoking increases the risk of lung disease. It's extra hazardous if you work with solvents.

Solvents, by their very nature, can never be anything but "two-faced"—useful, but also treacherous. Learn and follow the rules that should be posted at your workplace for handling and storing organic solvents. And remember:

1. Avoid breathing the vapors.
2. Wash off spills and splashes on the skin.
3. Don't smoke around solvents.
4. Practice good personal hygiene.

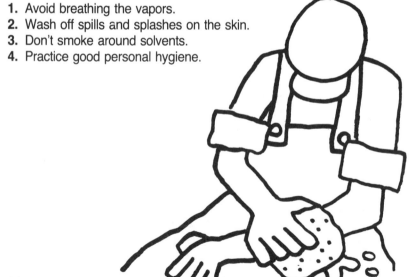

Formaldehyde: Risks & Safeguards

Formaldehyde, a potential cause of occupational cancer, is an especially troublesome substance because American industry uses so much of it in so many different ways.

The annual U.S. production of formaldehyde is about 7 billion pounds. Half of it will be used to produce synthetic resins, such as urea-formaldehyde or phenol-formaldehyde. These resins are mainly used as adhesives in making plywood, fiberboard and particleboard. Urea-formaldehyde is used in various coating processes, in paper products and, until recently, in making foam for insulation.

Acetyl resins, made from formaldehyde, are used to mold plastic parts for automobiles, home appliances, hardware, and garden and sporting equipment. Are some of your clothes "shrink-proof" and "crease-resistant?" Does the tissue you use have "wet strength?" You can thank formaldehyde and some of its chemical next-of-kin for all these conveniences. Formaldehyde is even used in some medicines because it can make viruses, venoms and irritating pollens less toxic.

All these different uses for formaldehyde aren't meant to scare you away from using the products. The wide variety is listed simply to indicate how widespread the use of formaldehyde is in industry. It's the workers in those manufacturing situations who most need to be on the lookout for overexposure.

In April 1981, the National Institute for Occupational Safety and Health (NIOSH) issued a bulletin recommending "that formaldehyde be handled as a potential occupational carcinogen and that appropriate controls be used to reduce worker exposure." The recommendation was based on studies showing that exposure to formaldehyde could cause nasal cancer in laboratory rats and mice.

Most chemicals known to cause cancer are also capable of causing a change in the genetic material of cells. Scientists have known for a long time that formaldehyde can cause such mutation.

There are other adverse health effects associated with exposure to formaldehyde. Concentrations ranging from 0.1 to 5 parts per million parts of air (ppm) can produce burning, watery eyes and general irritation of the upper respiratory passages. At higher levels—10 to 20 ppm—there may be coughing, tightening of the chest, a sense of pressure in the head, and palpitation of the heart. Exposure to 50 to 100 ppm and above can cause serious injury, such as fluid in the lungs, inflammation of the lungs, or even death.

Inflammation of the skin (dermatitis) may suddenly appear after a few days of exposure to formaldehyde solutions or resins made from the chemical. The reddish, itchy reaction may show up on the eyelids, face, neck, scrotum, fingers, back of the hands, wrists, forearms or other parts of the body—particularly where they are rubbed by the clothing.

The U.S. Department of Labor's Occupational Safety and Health Administration (OSHA) has set acceptable air contamination standards for formaldehyde concentrations. These range from a time-weighted eight-hour average of 3 ppm to a 5 ppm ceiling during that time. A 10 ppm maximum during any eight-hour shift is acceptable for no longer than 30 minutes total during the shift.

There are four basic methods for limiting exposure to formaldehyde:

1. *Substituting a different material.* Using an alternative material with a lower potential health risk, if practical, is most effective. But the new material must be checked out thoroughly in advance to make sure it doesn't cause health problems of its own.

2. *Controlling the source.* Airborne concentrations can be controlled by enclosing the operation, perhaps in combination with a good exhaust ventilating system. It is important that the exhaust system be checked at least every three months—even sooner if production methods have been changed.

3. *Isolating the worker.* This sometimes can be done by using equipment that workers can operate from a control booth or room to avoid direct contact.

4. *Providing personal protective equipment.* Respirators, goggles, gloves, etc., may be used on a short-term, temporary basis—while better methods are being installed, for maintenance, or during emergencies. But personal protective equipment should never be used as the only means to prevent or minimize formaldehyde exposure during everyday operations.

PCBs Are Dangerous

If the P.C. Bees were a family living in your neighborhood, you'd want to avoid them like the plague. Lucky for you, they're not a human family living next door. But unfortunately, the chemical family of PCBs—short for polychlorinated biphenyls—does live in countless American neighborhoods. And you should avoid them like the plague.

The chief use of PCB is as a liquid in electrical capacitors and transformers. You may have seen those bulky devices, some of which may contain PCB, attached to the tops of utility poles. Other uses are as additives in extreme pressure lubricants used in hydraulic systems, vacuum pumps, and gas transmission lines. PCBs are also used as coatings for investment molds in foundries, and in carbonless copying paper.

PCBs went into commercial production in 1929. In 1976, the Environmental Protection Agency banned most production of the substance. But (and this is a big point when it comes to today's health risk) the ban does not affect equipment already containing PCB.

As a result of this, a residential neighborhood near San Francisco recently was contaminated when an electrical transformer malfunctioned and sprayed lawns and shrubs underneath with the toxic chemical. In another incident, fire in a waterfront storage shed containing old transformers sent up clouds of PCB-laden smoke, endangering firemen and spectators. Highway spills of PCB from old transformers in transit have also caused problems.

PCBs can enter the body in several ways. The substance can be drawn into the lungs by breathing air contaminated with PCB vapor, mist or particles. It can come in through the skin during contact with material containing PCB or liquid PCB. The liquid also may get into the eyes. It can invade the digestive system through PCB-contaminated food.

Health problems can come about through either short-term (acute) exposure, or long-term (chronic) exposure. Signs of acute exposure include vomiting, stomach pains, loss of appetite and fatigue. In many cases, workers who come in contact with PCB develop a severe skin problem called chloracne which consists of pustules and cysts. The condition can be disfiguring.

Chronic exposure to PCB can cause liver damage leading to other complications. Recently, PCB has been implicated in other long-term health problems including cancer. Animal studies indicate PCB as causing liver cancer and some human studies have shown increased levels of liver cancer among workers exposed to PCB.

Impotence and other reproductive problems are associated with PCB exposure. Women exposed to PCB while pregnant have delivered stillborns and infants with skin and eye problems.

The Occupational Safety and Health Administration (OSHA) has standards limiting worker exposure by inhalation and skin contact with PCBs. By law, workers are not permitted to be exposed to an air concentration greater than one milligram of PCB per cubic meter of air. In addition to the air standard, all workers who might have some skin contact with PCB must be provided with protective clothing.

The National Institute for Occupational Safety and Health (NIOSH) would like to see the air standard tightened up. It has recommended cutting the air standard by 1,000—to one microgram of PCB per cubic meter of air. What NIOSH is saying, in effect, is that workers shouldn't be exposed to any PCB, since its proposed standard is the lowest detectable level that can be monitored using standard industrial hygiene sampling techniques.

There are several precautions that should be followed in dealing with PCBs. All fixed operations where the substance can become airborne, particularly in operations using temperatures above 131 degrees Fahrenheit, should be totally enclosed and ventilated so there is no chance of mist or vapor escaping.

In the case of movable or emergency operations (spills, for example) workers should be provided with a complete range of protective devices. These would include:

• Full suits of protective clothing through which PCB cannot penetrate, as well as gloves, hair covers and shoe covers. Such impermeable covering will prevent skin contact with PCB and its absorption into the body.

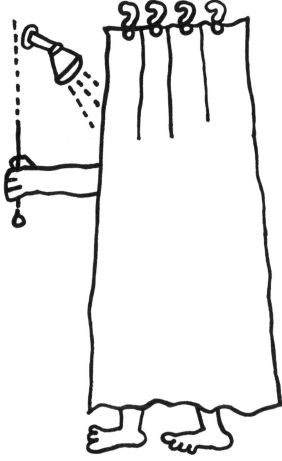

- Respiratory protection in the form of supplied-air respirators or self-contained breathing apparatus with a full facepiece, helmet or hood. The full facepiece, in addition to giving better respiratory protection, also provides protection to the face and eyes.
- Decontamination showers where workers can go directly after finishing the job. In the shower area, workers should deposit work clothing and respirators, wash and put on street clothing. Such a procedure can prevent the carrying of PCB on work clothes to the workers' cars and then into the homes where members of their families could be exposed.

The most common PCB compounds used today usually are light, straw-colored liquids which have chlorinated, aromatic odors. But they can also be in the form of clear yellowish oils or waxes. Your health, and that of your family, requires that you use every precaution to avoid contamination.

Handling Vinyl Chloride

Vinyl chloride (VC) is the basic ingredient in making polyvinyl chloride (PVC), which is used in more than half of all plastic products. The gas was generally considered to be of mild toxicity until January 1974, when vinyl chloride was found to cause a rare form of liver cancer called angiosarcoma, which cannot be detected until it is incurable.

Later studies showed that workers exposed to VC have higher than normal rates of cancer of the lung, brain and bone marrow. Vinyl chloride acts slowly. Symptoms of the cancers may not show up until 15 years or so after a worker's initial exposure.

In order to focus on the danger and the workers who are at risk, we need to understand the gas itself—the vinyl chloride—and the various production steps where it is used that are hazardous. The finished products made of polyvinyl chloride have not been proved hazardous, so far, in government and private laboratory tests.

That's good to know because polyvinyl chloride is all around us. You probably rode to work on a vinyl seat, walked across a vinyl-tiled floor on PVC-soled shoes, unwrapped vinyl from your lunch to eat on a vinyl tablecloth and relaxed to the sound of PVC records. At home, maybe the baby is content to suck on a PVC pacifier.

By the time the plastic reaches this finished-product stage, the vinyl chloride has been chemically locked into the PVC and will not come out again. The danger comes in the production process. Three basic steps are necessary to make vinyl products:

1. The vinyl chloride—or "monomer"—is produced in a closed process, usually involving a reaction between ethylene and chlorine.
2. Compressed to a liquified gas, the VC monomer is generally shipped to plants that produce the PVC resin. Here, batches of VC are "polymerized" in huge vats or reactors by the addition of catalysts. The PVC resins, after they are dried, are compounded with the further addition of plasticizers, stabilizers and lubricants. At this point, the resins may be converted to powders, pellets, pastes or film.
3. The PVC resins in their various forms, depending on products they are to be used in, are shipped to thousands of fabrication plants.

Workers at steps 1 and 2 face a variety of problems. There is the possibility of random leaks from pump seals, compressors, valves, gaskets and storage tanks. At both stages, workers have to deal with holding to a minimum the amount of gas that escapes during quality control sampling. Tank car workers may be exposed to high concentrations of the gas in the air during loading or unloading of the monomer.

Production of the basic monomer generally is an open-air operation and the concentration of the gas in the air is usually lower than at polymerization plants.

The riskiest occupation in the entire industry is that of vat cleaner. In this operation, workers have to climb into the polymerization vats or reactors and chip out the PVC residue. In its job health hazard series of pamphlets, the U.S. Department of Labor reports that, in the past, these cleaners have been surrounded to concentrations as high as 1,600 parts of VC per million parts of air. Reactor exposure levels have reached concentrations as high as 500 parts per million.

The main risk at the fabricating end, although much smaller than the earlier risks, can come from the small amount of gas that may not have been chemically locked into the PVC. This gas could leak during handling or processing. Heating increases this potential danger, as in extruding PVC resin around an electrical wire.

The best protection against vinyl chloride poisoning is prevention of gas leakage into the air. This a matter of engineering controls. The Occupational Safety and Health Act (OSHA) places the responsibility on employers. The law also requires strict monitoring of exposure levels, regular medical examinations, and long-term record-keeping.

Pesticide Poisoning

Farm work has become one of the nation's most hazardous occupations, particularly in those states with extensive commercial agriculture.

The reason: exposure to pesticides. California farm officials report that agriculture has a higher rate of injury due to toxic chemicals than any other industry. These injuries account for 75 percent of the more than 1,000 occupational poisonings reported each year. People who mix and apply pesticides are the most frequently poisoned.

Even this high rate of occupational poisonings may not tell the full story when it comes to field workers. A few years ago, Dr. Ephraim Kahn of the California Department of Health Services wrote in the Journal of Occupational Medicine, "officially we hear of only a small fraction, possibly as little as 1 percent, of the pesticide illnesses in field workers."

State farm officials say that California doctors receive some 14,000 requests a year to treat pesticide poisoning. Most of these involve people exposed to pesticides in the home or garden. Many of them are young children. Persons who live and work in farm communities are also frequent victims of pesticide exposure.

But agricultural workers and those who live near the fields are not the only ones at risk from this widespread problem. Firefighters and police must deal with chemicals in emergency situations. Overturned tanker trucks, or fires in storage facilities are instances of potential poisonous contamination that can result in health problems.

There are simple precautions that can help to reduce the hazards when pesticides are being used on your property or in nearby fields.

Close the windows. Keep children, pets and playthings inside where spray will not land on them. Don't let children or pets play on pesticide equipment or in areas where the chemicals are stored. If you and your family are accustomed to getting fruits and vegetables directly from fields and orchards, always wash them before eating.

Containers can be particularly troublesome unless you use care. Never use old pesticide containers to hold drinking water. Never put leftover pesticides in empty pop bottles or other containers that children might be attracted to. Keep all pesticide containers away from children—even empty ones may be poisonous.

Clothing worn while spraying, or worn in sprayed fields, should never be washed with the rest of the family's clothing. Laundered clothing hung out to dry should be placed where spraying cannot reach it.

If you are working in a sprayed field or your own garden, don't carry lunch, a snack or a beverage with you. Don't eat or smoke in a sprayed area. That's a good way to transfer poison from plants or the air to the inner parts of your body.

All workers have the right to know what pesticides are being used on the crops they work with. It is the responsibility of the grower or farmer, crew chief or other supervisors to provide workers with this essential information. It is printed on the label describing the chemical, its toxicity, first-aid treatment and other information. Workers who have been refused this information should contact the regional office of the Environmental Protection Agency or a local legal service office.

One of the most important functions of the EPA is setting up "re-entry times"—a period of time that workers must wait before going back into fields that have been sprayed. This period usually ranges from 24 to 48 hours. For awhile, the same re-entry times set for adults were being used for 10- and 11-year-old farmworkers who harvest apples, strawberries and potatoes. Fortunately for the health of the children, these standards are being reviewed and adjusted.

Many scientists believe, and several courts have ruled, that children cannot be compared to adults when it comes to setting safe levels of pesticide exposure. For all ages, the best rule is that the least exposure is best if it cannot be avoided entirely.

Pesticides and the Environment

As World War II was winding down in the mid-1940s, we opened a new conflict. This time the enemy was insect pests—infinitely smaller, but far, far more numerous. The big guns we wheeled out were synthetic chemical pesticides. Farmers and gardeners thought science had found the ultimate weapon, the magical wipe-out for destroyers of crops and forests, lawns and gardens. But that V-Day was celebrated too soon. The pesticide war is far from won.

After more than 35 years of waging chemical warfare against insects, weeds and plant diseases, these pests still destroy about one-third of the crop production in this country. The portion lost to insects alone has doubled since 1945, although the use of chemicals designed to kill insects has increased 10 times during the same period.

Puzzled at first, agricultural scientists figured out why: The insecticides kill not only the insect pests, but wipe out the beneficial insects as well. These good guys play an important part in the natural order of things—they survive by eating the bad guys we want to get rid of. By eliminating these natural allies of ours, we have to take on their jobs ourselves. More chemicals have to be used to control the pests that are no longer kept in check by their insect foes and parasites. That's how the chemical insecticide warfare escalates.

Then another problem arose. After repeated sprayings, some insects develop resistance to chemicals and pass along this trait to their offspring. In a fairly short time, we are faced with a breed of "superbugs" who are resistant to a variety of pesticides.

One of the first examples of this occurred in the cotton belt. After World War II, growers found DDT to be a cheap and effective way to control the boll weevil. It took just 10 years for a hardier strain of bug to come along which was not susceptible to DDT. Cotton farmers switched to new types of chemicals. In time, the bugs outgrew them, too. Today, all of the major cotton pests in the United States are resistant to one or more insecticides.

And it's not just the bugs. Plant diseases also are developing resistance to pesticides.

There are also harmful side effects. In California, pesticide damage poses a serious problem for the state's beekeepers. Each year they lose one hive in 10 to pesticides, according to a recent report cited by the California Agrarian Action Project. This is a serious concern for farmers, too, because honeybee pollination is essential to the production of California seed, nut, fruit and vegetable crops.

Drifting herbicides is another problem. Weedkillers applied to rice fields have harmed prune trees and sugar beet fields. The chemical 2,4-D, used by grain farmers to kill weeds, can harm grape vineyards. California officials have found cases where this herbicide has damaged vineyards 15 miles downwind from where it was applied.

You don't have to live in an agricultural area, either, to be affected by drifting chemical sprays. Utilities, railroads and highway crews have long used herbicides to control weed growth along rights-of-way. A group called Citizens for Environmental Protection in West Virginia fought such spraying. The group contended that homes, schools and streams were being hit by drifting defoliants. A study done for the Environmental Protection Agency (EPA) several years ago found that between 10 and 60 percent of pesticides applied by air travel more than 1,000 feet from the target area.

The chain of pesticide exposure is long and composed of many links. Agricultural workers are directly exposed in mixing, loading or applying the chemicals. They may also come in contact with leaves or soil by entering fields too soon after spraying. Others in nearby fields may be exposed by the drift of the pesticides.

Poison on a worker's clothing can be taken into the home, exposing whole families. And pesticide runoff into ponds, streams and groundwater can lead to serious health problems for entire communities.

The health questions raised by the intensive use of chemical pesticides and herbicides stretches from the chemical factories to the fields, to the workers and their families, and ultimately to the supermarket and the corner grocery.

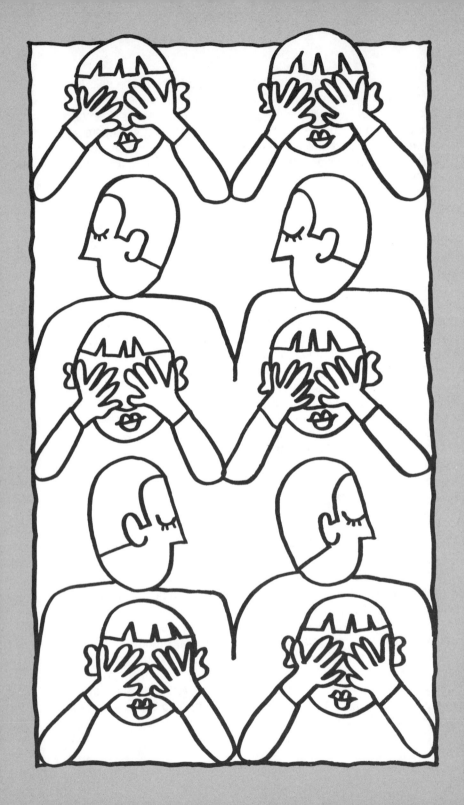

3 Physical Agents:

NOISE, LIGHT, HEAT, COLD, VISION, RADIATION & VIBRATIONS

Noise on the Job

Most workers tend to think of occupational hazards in terms of things they can see, smell, taste or touch: fumes, gases, liquid and solid toxic substances, machinery and so on.

But you can't apply these tests to one of the most widespread and potentially dangerous health hazards—noise. It surrounds us all the time at work, at play, even at rest. At excessive levels, it is a definite risk.

To understand this risk, it helps to know how your sense of hearing works. Sound begins as a vibration of the air. The air between you and the source of the sound is filled with particles too tiny to see. The vibration of the air agitates these particles into a wave-like motion. It is this motion—not the particles—that reaches your eardrum and makes it vibrate.

Beyond the eardrum are three tiny bones connected to each other. The "sound wave" that makes the drum vibrate also moves these little bones. The bones transmit the motion to a snail-shaped organ called the cochlea (Greek for snail) which is filled with liquid. The liquid passes the motion along to tiny hairlike structures or nerve endings. These hairlike cells change the motion to electrical energy, sending signals to the hearing center of the brain which interprets the sound.

This interpretation—the particular character of the sound—depends on the frequency of the air motion's ups and downs that reach the eardrum. Frequency is usually measured in cycles per second (cps). A frequency of 15 cps would be similar to the vibration of the lowest note on a church organ. A high whine from your TV might reach 15,000 cycles per second.

Just as frequency lets your brain know what range of sounds you are hearing from high to low, intensity measures the amount of agitated air reaching the eardrum which the brain interprets as volume or loudness.

The miracle of hearing takes place instantly. I have traced the various steps in detail to emphasize what a marvelously complex organ the ear is, and to suggest why such a sensitive apparatus needs to be protected against noise abuse.

The little hairlike cells that turn motion into electrical impulses can take just so much energy. Ordinarily, they ought to last you most of a lifetime. But if they are unduly agitated and overloaded by prolonged exposure to loud noises, they wear out before their time and your hearing suffers.

Noise intensity is measured on a decibel scale. There are several such scales, but the one most often used is the A scale because it most resembles human hearing. You will usually see the scale written as a number followed by dBA.

Here are some decibels and corresponding sounds: Using 0 as a reference level, 10 dBA would be the sound of rustling leaves; 30 dBA a ticking watch, and 60 dBA normal conversation. At 80 dBA, hearing damage can begin; 100 would be about the level of a food blender at two feet, or a circular saw, or the noise inside a construction plant. A level of 140 dBA—a jet with afterburner—can cause pain.

Exposure to industrial noises of 85 to 115 dBAs is not uncommon. Some work laws set an acceptable level of exposure for an eight-hour shift around the lower end of such levels. But studies have shown that exposure to 90 dBA for eight hours can cause serious hearing difficulties in one out of five workers, and one in 20 can be so severely affected that compensation is indicated.

Remember, the decibel scale is based on powers of 10 (logarithmic) and not on simple arithmetic. A reading of 10 dBA, for example, means that the sound is 10 times the reference sound. But 20 dBA doesn't mean that the sound is merely twice as loud as at 10, but 100 times as intense (10 x 10). A level of 30 dBA would be 1,000 times as loud (10 x 10 x 10) and so on.

As long as you remember that each additional 10 dBAs means the sound is increased tenfold, you won't be taken in by anybody who talks soothingly of "a few more decibels" as if they were counting apples. Each increase of 3 on the scale, for instance, represents a doubling of intensity. So 93 decibels is not "just over 90." It means that twice as much sound energy is pounding into your ear.

Noise: Enemy at Your Ear

Hearing loss—although the most noticeable and measurable—is just one of several possible adverse health effects of excessive noise. Prolonged exposure to loud noise is a source of stress. And the body reacts to noise stress in much the same way it responds to stress from any other cause: It seeks to protect itself from what the brain tells it is danger.

The blood vessels constrict in all organs except the muscles and brain. This tightening up is particularly noticeable in the intestines. The adrenal glands pour out more adrenalin which, in turn, increases the pulse rate, blood pressure and rate of breathing. The blood-clotting ability of the body rises. Extra fats may be released into the bloodstream.

These biological events are common reactions to stress from all sorts of causes, so we cannot say with certainty that noise alone is to blame. But this combination of body reactions, potentially, may dispose a person to heart disease and circulatory problems.

There is growing evidence that suggests a link between excessive noise exposure and the development and aggravation of an individual's tendency to disease. Commenting on the high incidence of heart disease in this country, William Stewart, a former surgeon general of the United States, said "the noise of 20th century living is a major contributory cause."

The idea that you can get used to noise is a myth. Constant racket may become such a part of the total environment that you may notice it less, or not at all. But you can't fool your body's response mechanism. It continues to react to loud noise as if danger were present, alerting you to action. This constant state of readiness, some researchers believe, could lead to so-called "diseases of adaption"—high blood pressure, headaches, asthma, ulcers and colitis.

Studies in noisy industries, for example, have shown that cases of ulcers were as much as five times as numerous as normally would be expected. Some animal studies point to the possibility that noise may be a risk factor in lowering human resistance to disease and infection.

Even the unborn are not safe from the possible ill effects of noise. While still in the mother's womb, the developing child responds to the sounds in the mother's environment. The mother's physical reaction to stress, whether caused by noise or some other circumstance, is also transmitted to the fetus. Stress has been shown to cause constriction of the uterine blood vessels which supply the developing child with nutrients and oxygen.

Noise has been linked with lower birth weights in a Japanese study of 1,000 births. The lower weights—under 5½ pounds, which fits the definition of prematurity—were also associated with lower levels of certain hormones believed to affect fetal growth. These studies do not tell us what levels of maternal noise exposure could potentially harm the fetus. But the findings are cause for concern.

It doesn't take a scientific study to tell you that noise and a good night's sleep don't go together. Noise can make it harder for you to fall asleep, wake you, or cause you to shift from deeper to lighter stages of sleep. This interference with sleep—the body's time out to let you recover from the day's demands—can take a toll on your health and general disposition.

An obvious and dangerous side effect of high noise levels, especially in industrial settings, is the diminished ability to communicate vocally. You may not be able to hear instructions or heed warnings that could be vital to your safety. In a study covering several industries, medical and accident records showed significantly higher reported accidents in noisier plant areas.

What can be done to eliminate or at least reduce the potential health hazards of noise? As is the case with most pollution (and noise is an environmental pollution), the best place to start is at the source.

Machinery can be designed or modified to run quieter. We read every day about some consumer product—cars, washing machines, fans— that are quieter. Is it asking too much to insist that industries show the same concern for the health and well-being of their workers?

If noise is caused by metal striking metal, something as simple as a thin film of polypropylene or a felt gasket might solve the problem. Vibration—a common source of noise—can be dampened by using spring mounts or shock-absorbing materials. Sound-absorbing ceilings and floor coverings may also help.

Distance is an effective sound-reducer. Noisy machines that can't be muted can be isolated, and possibly operated by remote control. And even the best-designed machinery can become noisy and dangerous if it isn't properly maintained.

Finally, there's personal protection—the least satisfactory method of noise-suppression because it doesn't get at the source of the problem and puts the burden on the individual worker. Earmuffs are best, followed by individually molded ear plugs. But even the best of these de-

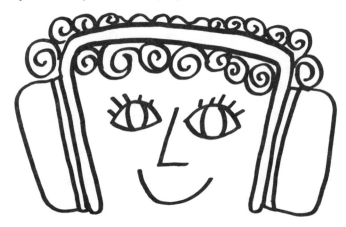

vices are often uncomfortable, especially in hot environments. Some workers have developed a fungus infection from keeping their ears covered for long periods.

Workplace Radiation—I

Radiation is generally divided into two categories—ionizing and non-ionizing. This is about non-ionizing radiation. But first, what's the difference between the two?

Ionizing radiation is the kind whose rays pack so much energy that when they interact with atoms they shatter them, remove electrons from them and cause them to develop an electric charge. A charged particle is an ion, so the force behind this charge is called ionizing radiation.

Ionizing radiation is that part of the energy band, or spectrum, that corresponds to X rays, alpha, beta and gamma rays, and neutrons. With their atom-smashing potential, when these rays ionize atoms in the body, they can damage them seriously, even fatally.

Non-ionizing radiation doesn't have enough energy to ionize atoms, so it is called non-ionizing. But it can still cause painful reactions as anybody can tell you who ever got sunburned from the ultraviolet rays of the sun, or suffered eye damage from the infrared heat of a furnace or other industrial heat source. Microwave ovens, radar, some medical apparatus and laser beams also use this end of the radiation band.

Here are some industrial exposures to various kinds of non-ionizing radiation and their major effects. This list is from *Work Is Dangerous to Your Health,* a handbook on health hazards in the workplace, by Jeanne M. Stellman, Ph.D., and Susan M. Daum, M.D. (New York: Vintage Books, 1973):

ULTRAVIOLET. Sunlight (all outdoor workers), electric-arc welding, germicidal lamps, "black light" used in blueprinting, laundry-mark identification, dial illumination. Ultraviolet radiation irritates and damages eye tissue; can cause painful sunburn and possibly skin cancer.

LASERS. Used in construction industry as reference lines, in medicine for surgery, in communications, in holography; may be used in drilling or wherever a concentrated high-energy beam is useful. Lasers are extremely hazardous to the eyes because the lenses of the eyes focus the light intensely on the retina.

INFRARED. Given off by all heated sources. Welders, steelworkers and glassblowers are exposed. Also used for drying and baking paint, varnishes and enamels. Infrared can cause damage to parts of the eyes. Workers may develop a condition known as "heat cataract."

MICROWAVES. Found in military, radio navigation, radar communications, food ovens, certain drying processes, medical diathermy. Eyes and testicles are most susceptible to damage; genetic effects and effects from long-term low levels are unknown. Microwave generators may also give off X rays.

RADIOFREQUENCY WAVES (RF). Used in heating equipment and for hardening metals, soldering and brazing. RF can be used in woodworking for bonding, laminating and gluing. This form of radiation is also used for sterilizing containers, thermo sealing and curing plastics. Improper operation or installation of equipment generating this form of radiation can lead to electrical shock and burns. If operator has wet feet, he or she can be electrocuted.

The key word for protection against non-ionizing radiation (any radiation, for that matter) is "shielding." Keep the rays from striking the body. This can mean anything from clothing to creams that screen out the sun, to reflective surfaces or the appropriate shade of the lens in welders' goggles.

Ovens and other sources of infrared (heat) radiation can be shielded with shiny materials to reflect the heat back toward its source. Some installations use a water screen for the same purpose.

Infrared radiation does not penetrate below the superficial layer of the skin. Its only effect is to heat the skin and the tissues immediately below it. The effects of ultraviolet waves is much more violent and a severe burn can be suffered, often before you know you have had too much exposure.

Microwaves penetrate deeply into the body and cause its temperature to rise. If the intensity of the microwaves is great enough, it can lead to permanent damage to the affected area. This deep heat penetrating ability is why the testicles are susceptible to damage. To function properly, the testicles have to maintain a temperature lower than the rest of the body. That's why they are on the outside. If this temperature rises because of microwave radiation, for example, the cell lining of the testicles can degenerate. Microwave sources can be effectively shielded by fine metal screens such as copper mesh, or thin steel plates.

With lasers, enclosure of the beam and remote-control operation are probably wise precautions. If this cannot be done, there are other safety steps that should be followed. Never align the beam by eye, or focus it on a mirror or other highly reflective surface. When the beam is aligned, it should be focused on a dull, non-reflecting object. Goggles should be worn that are designed for the particular kind of laser being used. The laser should be fixed-mounted so that it cannot be swung around accidentally.

Workplace Radiation—II

More than 770,000 American workers today are exposed to ionizing radiation on their jobs. You'll find them throughout industry—wherever there are X ray machines, radioactive materials, laser beams, certain electronic equipment and many other new tools and processes in use. That can cover a lot of ground, from aircraft factories to chemical plants, from mines to machine shops, from shipyards to steelworks—even the hospital and health care fields.

What is ionizing radiation and what can it do to your body?

Like everything else, radioactive materials decay over a period of time, often a very long time. But don't think of this decay as crumbling into dust. Radioactive decay is a process during which the element becomes more stable—that is, less radioactive. In doing this, the radioactive element shoots out particles and waves, moving at or near the speed of light. When these particles or waves strike atoms or molecules they tear them apart, leaving charged particles or ions. That's how we get the name "ionizing radiation."

The energy in this radiation is so high it can enter your body through the skin without you knowing it—like light passing through a pane of glass. That's called "external radiation hazard."

Ionizing radiation can also get into your body when chemicals containing radioactive materials are swallowed, inhaled, absorbed, or enter through open wounds. This is called "internal radiation hazard."

When ionizing radiation enters your body, it hits atoms and molecules with explosive force to form two potentially destructive chemical groups—oxidizing agents and free radicals. These chemicals are then free to attach themselves to any part of living cells and start doing their dirty work.

They break up proteins, destroy chromosomes, and change other chemicals of life. These chemical changes can affect the cell in a number of ways, causing:

- The death of the cell, either immediately or sooner than it might normally die;
- Change in the growth and division of the cell, ranging from no growth and division to uncontrolled growth and division (cancer);
- Permanent change in the way the cell works.

Since everything the body does is controlled by cells, it is conceivable that radiation can affect all functions of the body, including your thinking processes, muscular coordination, digestion, breathing, sight and sexual function.

There are three ways you can reduce external exposure to radiation—by limiting the time you're in a radioactive area, by putting as much distance as possible between you and the source, and by shielding yourself.

There are also three basic ways to minimize the internal hazard—by wearing protective clothing to keep the radioactive substance from getting on your skin where it can be absorbed, by using a respirator to keep from breathing it, and with engineering controls to stop the dangerous agents from becoming airborne in the first place.

While the hazards of radiation have been known for more than a century—and many workers sickened and died from exposure because too little was known at the time about its effects—unfortunately some modern workers aren't much better off.

It is important for workers who may be at risk to have a good understanding of ionizing radiation. With this information, they can make informed decisions about the level of exposure they are willing to accept.

An excellent booklet on this subject, called *Ionizing Radiation—A Guide for Workers*, has been written by Daniel Volz, an industrial hygienist. It is published by the Western Institute for Occupational/ Environmental Sciences, Inc., 2520 Milvia St., Berkeley, Calif. 94704.

Health Risks in Today's Office

If you've been working a few years, you probably can remember when it was fairly common for employers—and even some workers—to divide labor according to sex: "A man's job," "women's work," and so on.

That old-fashioned notion is fading fast as more and more women take their rightful places throughout the workforce. Still, some people cling to the myth that clerical, service and health care jobs, among others, are somehow cleaner, quieter and safer than other types of work. "Women's work," in other words.

It simply isn't true. Modern machines, new products—many chemically based—and radically changed working conditions have blasted this complacency. Women workers in the so-called clean-quiet-safe occupations face numerous and dangerous on-the-job risks.

According to figures compiled by the U.S. Bureau of Labor Statistics, hospitals are among the most dangerous places to work. Hospitals, traditionally, have been one of the largest employers of women. Slips, falls, sprains and physical injuries caused by lifting are among the occupational hazards faced by hospital workers, whether they be nurses, technicians or room and hallway cleaners.

Chemical hazards such as formaldehyde, anesthetic gases and bacteriocides make many hospital jobs dangerous, affecting porters as well

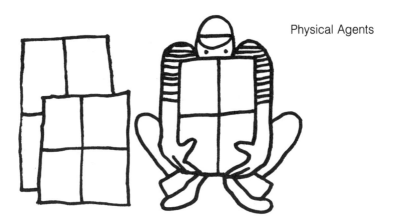

as surgeons. Numerous studies have pointed to the possible danger of low-level radiation from X rays and nuclear medicine procedures.

Office work, a kind of catch-all phrase that now covers a wide variety of job skills, is not the safe haven for women it once was thought to be. The clatter of office background noises, endured steadily for several hours, has the potential for impairing the hearing of secretaries and typists, as well as contributing to stress with its adverse effects on health.

The office environment can be contaminated in other ways. In older buildings, particles of asbestos from the lining in decaying air conditioning ducts can become airborne. When these microscopic asbestos fibers are inhaled, they can lodge in the lungs where they can cause cancer and other serious diseases up to 10 to 40 years later. Even in newer buildings, office remodeling can scatter asbestos fibers from acoustical tile and wallboard.

New buildings, in fact, can be even worse for employees' health. Many of these newer structures are tightly sealed for energy efficiency. But keeping air from leaking out also means keeping fresh air from getting in. Many air conditioning systems change the air only about once in 10 hours. As a result, noxious fumes from cigarette smoke, office equipment and even from some materials used in the construction are recirculated for long periods of time.

A study by the National Institute for Occupational Safety and Health (NIOSH) showed that a simple duplicating machine can give off methyl alcohol vapors in concentrations up to nearly four times the recommended exposure limits. This can cause nausea, dizziness, blurred vision and skin problems.

Technological innovations in office work often lead—as they do in "men's jobs"—not only to speed-up, but also to health problems. A prime example of this is the experience of women workers with video display terminals (VDTs). These machines, which look like a typewriter keyboard with a small television screen above it, are now used by many businesses such as newspapers, insurance companies, airlines and brokerage houses.

Workers who operate VDTs have complained of eyestrain, aching muscles and fatigue. Questions also have been raised about radiation hazards that may be caused by the terminals.

In a heartening example of union effectiveness, several unions in California, representing large numbers of women, formed the "VDT Coalition." This organization was instrumental in successfully urging NIOSH to conduct an evaluation of health risks in working with the machines. As a result, NIOSH developed recommendations for redesign of work stations, control of screen glare, mandatory rest breaks and eye tests.

Unions in the coalition include San Francisco-Oakland Local 52 of The Newspaper Guild, the Communications Workers of America, the Office and Professional Employees International Union, the Graphic Arts International Union, and the United Transportation Union.

The 'Electronic Sweatshop'

What's the fastest growing high-risk occupation? Astronaut? Nuclear plant janitor? Junk food tester?

No. In terms of the number of people involved, and in the dizzying range of hazards they are exposed to, office workers today probably make up the fastest growing high-risk occupational group. Ironically, the dangers have come about largely through technologies that were supposed to make clerical work easier, cleaner and more attractive:

- Tightly sealed, box-like buildings to keep out dust and annoying street noises and fumes, but which succeed mostly in trapping all the bad air inside.
- Photocopying machines to end the messy, tiresome chore of making carbons or cutting stencils, but which can give off ozone gas that irritates eyes, nose, throat and lungs.
- Automation, that magic genie to let us get more done faster, smoother and with less hassle, but through which, in the words of Working Women Education Fund, "the enjoyable aspects of clerical work—variety, contact with other people, natural rest breaks and changes in routine—are threatened with elimination. The most stressful aspects—repetitive tasks, constant sitting, dead-end jobs, a relentless fast work pace—are on the rise."

Not only are the health hazards rising as newer machines and demands are introduced, but the numbers of clerical workers exposed to the risks also are increasing.

Clerical workers already have replaced manufacturing workers as the single largest segment of the workforce. In the 1980s, more than half of all new jobs will be white collar. And, in another 30 or 40 years, some crystal-ball gazers predict that from 80 to 90 percent of the entire workforce will be in jobs involving information processing.

Women, who still fill most of the office jobs, are particularly vulnerable to the growing hazards. Not only are they likely to be in the most highly regimented jobs with the greatest stress, but they bear the heaviest home responsibilities as well.

Here are a few of the office hazards; how they can adversely affect health, and what can be done to eliminate or reduce the risks:

VDTs. Video display terminals (VDTs), now almost as commonplace in many offices as typewriters, can cause eyestrain, temporary color blindness, headache, tension and pain in the neck and back. These machines also give off low levels of ionizing radiation and radio frequencies which might have the long-term potential of damaging the genes. Frequent rest breaks can reduce the harmful effects of VDTs on vision. Screens should be adjustable to minimize glare and the strain of sitting for long periods.

Photocopying machines. The photocopy machine is also such a familiar part of the office scene that most workers tend to forget that it can be a source of health hazards. These include the chemicals used in the toners and in the fusing process, high intensity light, ozone and the electrical circuitry.

The powdered form of dry toners usually contain carbon black, polymers (plastics), and organic dyes. Wet toners contain a liquid solvent. Both have been known to cause skin rashes and allergic skin reactions among operators. These reactions also have been caused by the chemicals used in the coated paper. Workers who develop rashes after handling toners or papers should avoid such contact, wearing rubber gloves if necessary. Workers can also be exposed to chemicals by inhaling vapors and dust emitted during operations of the machines.

High voltage used to produce the intense light required in the copying process can change oxygen to ozone gas. The pungent smell is sometimes described as an "electrical odor." Low doses of ozone can cause eye, nose and throat irritation. Higher doses may result in coughing, choking, fatigue, pain or pressure in the chest. While most machines do not produce ozone above the OSHA threshold of 0.1 parts per million (ppm), machines that are serviced infrequently and are poorly maintained may exceed the limit. If you can smell the odor, the concentration is near or above the level you should avoid. Photocopiers should always be located in well-ventilated areas.

Noise. Noise adds another complication to the office environment. Electric typewriters, tabulators and addressing machines have been measured at 80 decibels (dBA) or higher. For comparison, some scientists believe a dBA range in the mid-60's is comfortable, and set a threshold of 85 dBA before hearing problems could appear. The OSHA limit is 90 dBA exposure for eight hours. Prolonged exposure to high noise levels has been linked to circulatory, digestive, neurological and psychological problems.

High tech created these problems in the pursuit of productivity and profits. The same ingenious know-how needs to be applied just as diligently in the pursuit of workers' health and safety. Organized workers and responsible manufacturers and managements can combine to put an end to what has been aptly called "The Electronic Sweatshop."

Health Problems Created by VDTs

Probably no piece of equipment is changing office work more today than the video display terminal, or VDT. These machines have a television-type screen above a keyboard that displays information. There are more than 3 million of them in use now and a million more probably will come on line soon. They are used widely by government and private industry; in publishing, communications, banking and insurance; by computer operators and airline reservations clerks. They are also sometimes called CRTs—for cathode ray tubes.

Whatever you call them, these machines operate the same way your television set does. A cathode, or electron gun, beams electrons at an anode, the tube screen, where they cause phosphors to give off colored lights to produce an image.

VDTs may release low, but potentially dangerous, levels of radiation including X rays, microwaves and/or ultraviolet and infrared lights. Some testing has been done by government and industry, with mixed results. Union and health specialists have challenged the findings. Much more needs to be done in this area of research.

This section will focus on the everyday physical and mental effects on workers who use VDTs. The most common complaints are eye strain, sore neck and back muscles, headaches and stress, usually in combinations because they are related.

Much of the following information is based on a booklet published by the New York Committee for Occupational Safety and Health (NY-COSH), an organization of workers, unions, and health and legal professionals in the New York City area.

Eyes have three main sets of muscles. One set moves the eyes up and down and from side to side. Another adjusts the size of the pupils to varying light intensities. Another, the ciliary muscles, changes the shape of the lenses to bring objects being viewed into focus. When eyes are focused at close range, the ciliary muscles must compress the lenses, squeezing them down. After viewing something at close range for a long time, like a VDT screen, these muscles get very tired. A good work rule for VDT operators would provide a 15-minute break every hour, or a half-hour break every two hours. The rest period should be spent in an open area, away from the machines, to rest the eyes by viewing at a greater distance.

Glare is a significant cause of eye strain. This can come from two main sources: glare on the VDT screen itself, from windows, shiny work surfaces, keyboards and lighting that is too bright or poorly located in relation to the machines, or from a background that is too bright, such as windows or white walls.

Some operators put cardboard visors above the screen or to the side. There is nothing wrong with such makeshift devices, but it is a better long-term solution to persuade the employer of the importance of correct equipment and workplace design. Sunglasses are not recommended. They may improve viewing temporarily, but they may pose greater long-term hazards to the eyes.

Operators who wear corrective eyeglasses, particularly bifocals, often have special eye problems as well as posture problems. If necessary, these workers should be fitted with special lenses designed to focus at the normal viewing distance from the eyes to the screen. In the case of bifocals, the lower part of the lenses is designed for reading at a distance of about 12 inches. This means the wearer can only focus by leaning forward and tilting the head backward, putting a strain on neck and back muscles.

The problems of tired eyes and sore muscles can be further aggravated by overall stress. Working with VDTs is a demanding job, often requiring intense concentration. Workers who must provide information from the VDT screen to the public—sometimes irate and unsympathetic—are caught in a squeeze between the customer and the machine. Some machines are so set up that supervisors can directly monitor an operator's work, another source of stress. All of these factors can have a multiplying effect. Tired people have a harder time handling stress; stress makes you tired, and so on.

VDTs are here to stay. If there are problems—and there probably are—the first step in correcting them is learning how to recognize and evaluate the health hazards. Make a list, form a committee (or better, work through the union health and safety committee) and work it out with the employer.

Good Lighting in the Workplace

Of all the things that can affect your comfort, safety and efficiency at work—noise, odor, space, temperature among others—lighting probably is the single most important. The reason for this is simple: 85 percent of the information we get from our surroundings is perceived through the eyes. And the eyes can't do the job well if the light is bad.

Lighting can even affect your mood—how you feel on the job, your sense of wellbeing. Think for a moment about how you respond to an overcast day.

The Women's Occupational Health Resource Center (WOHRC) at the Columbia School of Public Health in New York lists four fundamental factors in visibility as they apply to various aspects of a task and the surroundings. These are time, size, contrast and brightness.

Time is especially important if you're working with moving machinery. You have to be able to see quickly; there's no way to stop the machine for a longer look. So the lighting must be adequate for quick, accurate visibility.

Size becomes important if you're working with small parts. The light must be adequate to see details.

Contrast is critical between the task you're doing and the background. Anybody who has ever darned a black sock with black thread can get the point—usually the needle in the tip of the finger.

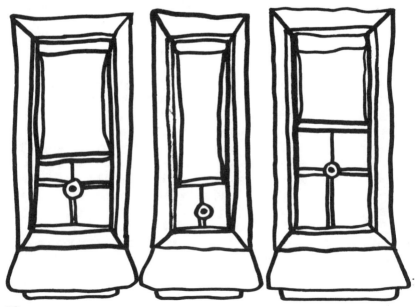

Of all these factors, brightness is the most controllable. By putting more light on a task, we can increase visibility in spite of lack of time to see well, small size or poor contrast.

A good lighting level may vary for a particular operation, depending on the characteristics of individual workers. Older workers, for example, need more light. The amount of light reaching the retina decreases with age. We also become less resistant to glare as we grow older.

Glare usually results from light in the wrong place. It can make seeing difficult, cause eye strain and fatigue, interfere with production and lead to accidents. Glare also can be reflected into the eyes from shiny surfaces. This can be a problem in many industrial operations involving such reflecting materials. Unless it is controlled as far as possible, this type of glare is particularly dangerous where moving machinery is involved.

Controlling glare, in many cases, is a matter of decreasing excessive brightness. Shielding of the light source also is important. Windows should have shades or blinds. Lighting equipment should be mounted so the light shines on the work rather than into the workers' eyes. Workers also should be positioned so that the bright lights do not come into their angle of vision. Shields in front of the lights can do this. An angle of 45 degrees for the shield is ideal.

Shadows pose other problems. A good way to avoid shadows is to have the light come from many different directions, rather than just one. In addition to different light sources, diffusion of lighting can be helped by using walls, ceilings and floors as reflecting surfaces. Light-colored, matte finishes are recommended.

Shadows may be desirable in some instances because they help our depth perception and viewing of details. This can be accomplished by supplementary lighting on the particular work at hand without interfering with the overall lighting.

Even though eyesight may seem automatic and effortless, it takes energy to see. When improper lighting makes the eyes work harder to see, you can become tired and irritable. The eyes may water and the eyelids redden. You may experience double vision or headache. There may be difficulty in focusing.

The Illuminating Engineering Society has published tables of lighting for most major seeing tasks. Your shop steward or safety committee will know about these studies. But you don't have to be an illuminating engineer to make a quick and easy spot check of a particular workplace. Pocket-type meters are available, usually for under $50.

A good maintenance program is essential to keep a lighting system up to its maximum efficiency. Over time, lamps can grow dim. Dirt can accumulate on fixtures and room surfaces.

Here are a few questions from a lighting checklist suggested by the Women's Occupational Health and Resource Center which you should keep in mind:

- Does the lighting in your work area create glare or shadows that make it harder for you to do your job?
- Do you feel you have to strain to see your work clearly? Do you bend over your work, squint, bring the work closer to your eyes?

If the answer to any of these is "yes," maybe you have a lighting problem that ought to be looked into.

Taking Care of Your Eyes

While you are reading these words, you probably are taking for granted one of the most remarkable things your body does for you: Performing the act of seeing. Most of us are like the fellow who returned from vacationing in the West and his friend asked: "Well, how did you find California?" The joker quipped: "Simple. I just opened my eyes and there it was."

But there's more to seeing than just opening your eyes. In the first place, you don't actually "see" with your eyes. You see with your brain. The eyes are simply very delicate and complex little TV-like cameras that direct light rays to the back of your eyeballs. This curved inner surface about the size of a postage stamp—the retina—contains about 130 million vision cells.

These cells collect and change the shifting patterns of light to impulses which are transmitted to the brain by the optic nerves. The brain translates these light impulses into the sensation of seeing, continuously, in the twinkling of an eye.

Like other organs and parts of the body, the eyes are subject to problems, caused by accidents or ailments. In either case, uncorrected eye problems can interfere with productivity, safety and comfort at work, school or home. Eye care is of two kinds:

1. Precautions—things you can do. Follow safety precautions, on the job or off, wherever there is the possibility of eye injury. The eyes are particularly vulnerable to flying particles (metal, stone, wood) thrown off by power equipment such as drills, cutting instruments and welding equipment. The eyes also can be harmed by irritating vapors or airborne particles. Safety eyewear always should be provided in such work situations. Use it, by all means. Another point to remember: 45 percent

of vision-impairing accidents happen around the home, according to the National Society to Prevent Blindness. The same precautions apply as for on-the-job hazards.

2. Treatment—things you should have an eye care specialist do for you. Eye ailments should be treated immediately to prevent any loss of sight. If you should experience any of the following symptoms, see a specialist at once: Sudden loss of vision. Flashes of light. A feeling that a curtain or veil is being pulled down in front of your eyes. Persistent or sudden severe pain or discomfort in the eyes.

One of the common eye ailments is "pink eye" or conjunctivitis. Although some people associate pink eye with childhood, it is not something to kid around with. It can show up as swollen, puffy eyelids that itch or burn, possibly with a discharge. Common causes are bacterial or viral infections, allergies (including allergies to make-up), and eye injuries. Pink eye can be contagious and spread through physical contact. If you have pink eye, you should get medical care to prevent more serious infection.

The two eye diseases most associated with adults over the age of 40 are cataracts and glaucoma. Glaucoma is a condition of increased pressure inside the eyeball. It is usually painless and can develop over a long period of time without your knowing it. Unfortunately, by the time you notice something is not right with your vision, permanent damage usually has occurred. Your eye care specialist can easily and painlessly measure the pressure inside the eyeball, as well as check for changes in the field of vision and in the internal structure of the eye.

Tell your eye care specialist if anybody in your family has glaucoma because the tendency to develop the condition can be inherited. Early detection and treatment can prevent blindness.

Cataracts are more common among people past the age of 55, although in rare cases they can occur at birth. Cataracts also can be caused at any age by accidents or disease. The first sign is a blurring of the vision. The condition progresses slowly and painlessly as the lens of the eye becomes increasingly cloudy. Cataracts cannot be cured by medication, but the cloudy lens can be removed surgically. After cataract surgery, when the eyes are completely healed, eyeglasses or contact lenses are prescribed to replace the clouded lenses that have been removed.

Vision care is provided by three types of professionals:

Ophthalmologists (licensed Doctor of Medicine, M.D.) are physicians who specialize in diagnosing and treating eye diseases, and perform eye surgery. They also test eyes for defects and prescribe corrective lenses.

Optometrists (licensed Doctor of Optometry, O.D.) test the eyes for vision defects and prescribe corrective lenses or therapy. Their training also qualifies them to detect eye conditions or diseases which may need to be referred to an ophthalmologist or another physician.
Opticians fill prescriptions written by ophthalmologists and optometrists. The optician's role also includes helping you order the size and shape of the frames for your eyeglasses and in providing a proper and comfortable fit.

The miracle of sight is not something to be taken for granted. With care against injury on your part, and prompt seeking of specialized help when you need it, your eyes can continue to perform their remarkable function.

Indoor Pollution Hazards

When you hear the words "air pollution," what's the first thing you think of? Smog? Smokestacks belching visible pollutants? Acid rain?

The big outdoors. That's where most people think air pollution lurks to endanger our health. But indoor air pollution may hold the greater danger of serious health problems, according to a report to Congress by the General Accounting Office (GAO).

Higher concentrations of air pollutants have been found in indoor environments than outside, the GAO says, adding that people normally spend 70 to 80 percent of their time indoors.

Ironically, the problem may be getting worse because we are trying to do something good—save energy. As more and more industries, businesses, offices and homes try to cut down on energy consumption by sealing up the nooks and crannies where heat can leak out, they may be trapping air pollutants generated inside, causing the levels of concentration to rise.

Indoor pollution can come from a number of sources. Carbon monoxide can be generated by gas appliances, leaking furnaces, automobiles in attached garages, chimneys and the like.

Radon, a radioactive gas, is a natural substance produced by the decaying of radium. It can build up inside buildings from construction materials, or from soil and rock formations underneath. The concentration can increase in structures where there is little fresh air coming in. Lengthy exposure to radon in concentrations higher than those in the outside atmosphere can increase the risk of lung cancer.

Formaldehyde is another substance that can be emitted into the indoor environment through building materials, insulation, furniture, textiles and other products. Preliminary studies have shown that formaldehyde can cause cancer in rats. In Massachusetts, more than 100 persons were hospitalized with acute health complaints traced to formaldehyde foam insulation.

Asbestos is a notorious carcinogen—a cancer-causing agent. And although its use was banned in certain building construction in 1973, it still is found in existing older structures. The yearly rate of asbestos production actually is increasing. It continues to be used in many products because of its heat-resistant properties.

Asbestos particles, as well as dust, soot, ash or cigarette smoke can be harmful because they are so tiny. They can go through the respiratory system and be deposited in the lungs. Asbestos-related diseases can take 10 to 40 years to develop.

Nitrogen dioxide levels higher than the federal standard have been found in homes with gas stoves, according to a study by the Harvard School of Public Health.

All of these hazards add up to one problem that is bigger than is recognized by federal agencies, the GAO says. The reason for this, as reported to Congress, is that no federal agency feels it has a mandate to safeguard the air anywhere except in the workplace.

This singleminded approach can put different agencies—each doing what it sees as its main job—on a collision course. For example, the Environmental Protection Agency (EPA) claims that if the Department of Energy's conservation program of lowering air exchange were applied across the board to every home in America, cancer deaths would increase by 10,000 to 20,000 a year.

As one possible way out of this dire cross-purpose result, the General Accounting Office recommends that EPA be given a mandate for protecting air quality in the non-workplace.

There are other useful ways that could be explored. European countries have been studying indoor air pollution for years, and they have found that controlling the quality of products is one of the most effective and enforceable corrective measures.

The GAO also says that research is needed to establish the long-term effects of indoor pollution and its interaction with other health factors. Beyond this, the agency says that the public needs to be better informed about what can be done to lower indoor pollution. This information could include ways of airing out the home, and cutting off emission sources, such as sealing off asbestos.

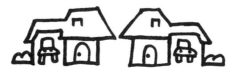

How Odors Affect You at Work

Can something you can't hear, see, taste or touch affect your health and your work? Yes, indeed, if that "something" is odor.

Although generally underrated, odors—both pleasant and offensive—play a significant role in occupational safety and health. Pleasant smells can induce a sense of well-being, stimulate your appetite, enhance the quality of an environment, and increase your productivity on the job.

Even unpleasant odors can perform a useful function by warning you of the presence of toxic substances. For instance, it is not just by chance that natural gas has a distinctive smell, or that insecticides aren't made to smell like vanilla.

On the other hand, bad smells can produce a wide range of adverse effects. Researchers have linked offensive odors with nausea, headache, loss of appetite, sleeplessness, impaired breathing, even allergic reactions. Foul smells also have been associated with irritability and depression.

From an economic standpoint, persistent offensive odors can stifle the growth and development of areas that are affected. Both labor and industry naturally tend to avoid places with uncontrolled odor problems. This has an obvious effect on jobs and payrolls. Several methods of controlling odors have been used successfully. These include combustion, absorption, adsorption, dilution, counteraction, masking, containment, etc.

Hydrocarbons turn to odorless carbon dioxide and water when subjected to heat at around 1,200 degrees Fahrenheit. Sulfur and nitrogen compounds become sulfur oxides and nitrogen oxides. However, the

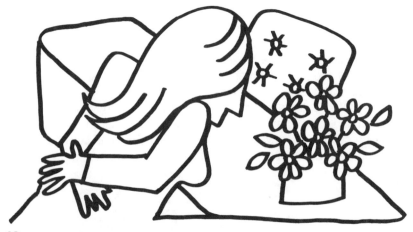

combustion must be complete. Partial combustion can make a smelly problem worse by forming malodorous aldehydes.

If odorants are soluble in water or some other liquid, absorption may be a solution. A spray of water, for example, can absorb the smell of ammonia in the air.

Although the word looks similar, adsorption works in an entirely different way. In adsorption, the odor-causing compounds are gathered into the surface of a solid. One of the best and widely used adsorptive materials is activated charcoal. Charcoal is particularly useful because it has the ability to adsorb so many types of substances under almost all conditions.

If an odorant is diluted below the "threshold concentration"—the point where your nose tells you it is offensive—the environment will become odor-free.

When certain odors are smelled together, they tend to cancel each other, or certainly diminish the smell of each. Among such counteractant pairs are cedarwood and rubber, balsam of Tolu and wax, paraffin and rubber.

In some cases, a disagreeable-smelling compound can be changed to something non-odorous or less unpleasant by chemical oxidation. The odorants in a scrubbing solution, for example, can be oxidized by the addition of chlorine or potassium permanganate. Acetic acid combined with ammonia produces ammonium acetate. Ultraviolet radiation will also result in chemical conversion of some odorants to compounds with less offensive odors.

Some situations may call for containment to reduce the emission of odors. Fuel tanks, sewage ponds and other open storage areas often require no more than covers, although containment doesn't get at the source of the odors.

Offices and other small work areas can often be kept odor-free by a well-designed and maintained air conditioning system with humidity controls. Chemical deodorizers for office use may have some degree of odor-masking properties. But they should also have disinfectant properties as well for floors, walls, closets, drains, wash basins and toilet bowls.

Heat Stress in a Hot Workplace

Millions of Americans work in hot, humid environments—from mines to smelters; from bakeries to laundries. All of them run the risk of heat stress. The body has to work harder to keep its internal temperature within safe limits when the heat of the workplace approaches or rises above that of normal body temperature, 98.6 degrees Fahrenheit.

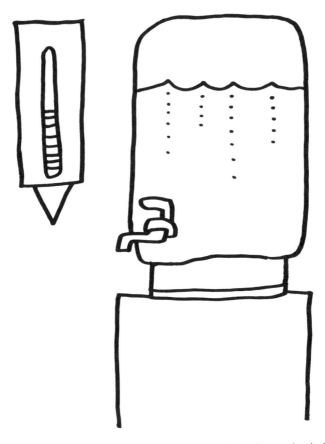

A part of the brain acts as a thermostat, keeping tabs on body heat and sending out signals to the cooling system. The heart pumps more blood. The tiny vessels (capillaries) near the surface of the skin go into action, radiating heat into the atmosphere. At the same time, water seeps through the skin in the form of sweat and evaporates with a cooling effect.

But when the space around you is nearly as hot or hotter than the body's normal temperature, this automatic system can become stressed. The signals still go out from the brain. But the blood brought near the surface cannot transfer the heat if the outside air and the blood heat are nearly in balance. The release of fluid through the skin and sweat glands becomes almost the only way of maintaining constant body temperature. But the only cooling effect of sweat is by evaporation. And if the environment itself is heavy with moisture—high humidity— evaporation is reduced.

All this rushing around of the blood toward the surface cuts down on the amount going to the active muscles. Strength declines. Fatigue comes on sooner. The brain may not act as sharply as it ordinarily would in doing detailed work or retaining information.

Common hazards include heat stroke, heat exhaustion and heat cramps. Heat stroke is a serious medical emergency, requiring quick action. Untreated, it can be fatal. The disorder can be recognized by elevated body temperature; hot, dry skin with red or blue splotches, mental confusion, fainting, or coma. First aid should begin at the first sign of heat stroke by immediately removing the victim to a cool area and soaking the clothing with cold water. Summon an ambulance and, while waiting for medical help to arrive, fan the victim vigorously to increase cooling.

Heat exhaustion, or heat collapse, is a common disorder and comes on quickly. Characteristically, the victim may feel weak, dizzy, nauseated or faint. Unlike heat stroke, the victim's skin may be cool and clammy with an ashen-gray color. Body temperature remains normal and pupils of the eyes are dilated. Generally, the symptoms are relieved quickly when the victim is moved to a cool area. When there is severe dehydration—a rare occurrence—hospitalization may be necessary.

Heat cramps are painful muscle spasms affecting the muscles of the arms, legs and stomach. These happen most often in workers whose salt intake does not replace what they lose through excessive sweating. The cramps often can be relieved rapidly by drinking a dilute solution of salt water. This can be made easily by dissolving half a teaspoon of table salt in a gallon of water. But a note of caution: If you have high blood pressure, or are on a low sodium diet, or taking diuretics, consult your physician about the hot environment you work in and the wisdom of taking salt. Do this before the emergency arises.

If you work in a hot environment, there are several things you can do to minimize the risks:

1. Make sure you drink enough water to equal the amount of sweat produced. A worker can lose up to three gallons of fluid a day through sweating.
2. Dress properly for the environment you work in. Unless special protective clothing is required, you should wear as little clothing as possible. It should be loose fitting and, preferably, made of 100 percent cotton to help evaporation.
3. Make sure that at least one worker in the area knows the signs and symptoms of heat disorders and appropriate first aid measures.

Certain groups of people have a greater risk than others of developing complications related to heat stress and should avoid working in hot environments. Among these are the elderly, pregnant women, diabetics, alcoholics, and people with heart disease, sickle-cell anemia or arteriosclerosis. Drug use also can be a risk factor. If you are taking prescription or over-the-counter medication and work in a hot environment, consult your physician or pharmacist.

Employers can help by allowing workers to get used to heat gradually. This may take a week or longer. The physical changes that take place in the body during this acclimatizing process can minimize the strain of adjusting. But remember, it may take a few days to get used to the heat all over again after a leisurely vacation or extended illness.

Heat disorders are serious. The hazards can be indoors at any time of the year, or outside under the hot summer sun. But knowing how to spot them quickly, and knowing what to do about relieving them, can help to safeguard your health and well-being and that of your co-workers.

Coping with Cold Weather Work

Cold is an occupational hazard year-round for thousands of workers in packinghouses, freezer plants, cold storage and cold-test facilities. When winter settles in, they are joined by millions of outside workers who have to deal with cold as a job risk—construction and maintenance crews, police officers, fire personnel, postal workers, farmers, ranchers, lumberjacks and so on.

Severe cold can cause more than discomfort. It has the potential for inflicting serious injury. One of the more serious injuries is frostbite—freezing of the exposed tissue. In order of severity, frostbite may be:

- First degree—freezing without blistering or peeling.
- Second degree—freezing with blistering and peeling.
- Third degree—freezing with death of skin and possibly deeper tissues.

The most common targets of frostbite are the ears, nose, chin, fingers and toes. Usually, the first sensations are a prickling feeling, itching and numbness. In appearance, a frostbitten area first may become pale, then turn purplish, and finally black in severe cases as the tissue dies.

If you are out in the field, you can treat superficial frostbite—frostnip—by firm but gentle pressure of a warm hand, or by placing the affected fingers in the armpit. If the toes or heels are affected, footwear should be removed, the feet dried and rewarmed, then covered with dry socks or other protective footwear.

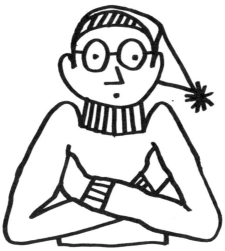

Rapid warming at temperatures slightly above body heat (98.6 degrees Fahrenheit) may help to reduce the danger of the tissues dying. You can do this by immersing the frozen area in water that feels warm to the normal hand—around 104 to 107.6 degrees Fahrenheit—but no warmer. The use of dry heat, such as an open fire or a stove, is not recommended because this kind of heat source is difficult to regulate.

A word of warning about an old wives' tale: Never try to treat frostbite by rubbing with snow! In fact, rubbing of any sort will only increase the damage. As with any injury, severe cases should be treated by your physician.

Another serious condition which must be treated promptly and properly is hypothermia—abnormally low body temperature. This condition can be brought about by prolonged exposure to atmospheric cold, or immersion in icy water. The risk of immersion is an obvious occupational hazard for fishermen, sailors and others who work on or around water in the winter.

In hypothermia, the internal (core) body temperature may range from around 95 Fahrenheit down to as low as 77 Fahrenheit. As the core temperature drops into the mid-90 degree range, the victim may become listless, confused, and make little if any effort to keep warm. At around 85 Fahrenheit, serious problems may appear, such as significant drops in blood pressure, pulse rate and respiration.

Mild hypothermia generally responds to a warm bed or a warm bath. Moderate to severe cases usually require more aggressive rewarming. But active rewarming is hazardous and should be undertaken only under medical supervision and with careful monitoring.

A less life-threatening cold disorder is urticaria, which can develop in hypersensitive individuals upon even limited exposure to cold wind. This condition—similar to hives—generally shows itself as a burning sensation of the skin about 30 minutes after exposure. If you are susceptible to this kind of cold affliction, precaution against exposure is your best course of action.

Probably the best advice to anybody who is exposed to cold—whether on the job or following your favorite winter sport—is summed up by the three "keeps" for keeping healthier and heartier in winter: Keep warm. Keep dry. Keep moving.

Controlling Hand and Wrist Damage

Of all the tools you use on the job, none are as delicate and complicated and as vulnerable to damage as your hands and wrists. These compact bunches of nerves, tendons, ligaments, blood vessels and bones are marvels of mechanical engineering. Carrying out the brain's bidding, they have fashioned every man-made object in the universe. But some of the things we ask them to do (especially to do over and over again) can cause trouble.

There are many occupations where a worker has to perform countless repetitive motions during the workshift. The factory assembly line is one of the most demanding worksites, and the United Auto Workers has produced an excellent guide called "Strains and Sprains" which describes problems faced by many of its members. Much of this article is based on the UAW's research.

Long-term damage to the wrists and hands—not counting such instant injuries as cuts, burns, bruises, etc.—is usually caused by one or more of the following job demands:

- Twisting hand movements, or bending of the wrist, repeated over long periods of time;
- Using the hands and wrists in an awkward position;
- Excessive pressure on parts of the hands and wrists;
- Vibration from tools and equipment;
- Exertion in combination with any of these activities or conditions.

Carpal Tunnel Syndrome can result from job operations that require a twisting motion of the hand, or a bent wrist. The median nerve passes through a channel in the wrist called the Carpal Tunnel on its way to supplying the thumb, index finger, middle finger and part of the ring finger.

Repeated excessive pressure on this nerve can cause numbness, a

98

burning or tingling sensation, shiny palm, a wasting of the muscles at the base of the thumb, and clumsiness in using the hands. The symptoms often are strongest at night. Sometimes only one side of the hand is affected.

Mild cases are relieved by wearing a wrist splint, usually at night, to provide a rest for the overworked wrist. More complicated treatment includes local injection of cortisone-type steroid drugs to relieve pain, or surgery as a last resort. But prevention, through the use of better designed tools and work practices, is better than treatment, as it is in most cases of job-related hazards.

Tendonitis is a condition in which the tendons become inflamed and sore because of overuse. Tendonitis is usually associated with operations that require repetitive motions. Symptoms include pain, swelling, tenderness and redness of the hands and wrists and, sometimes, even the forearms. Use of the hands and fingers can be greatly reduced.

Rest for the affected parts is the basis of effective treatment, possibly combined with heat and use of a splint. But, again, long-term relief depends on eliminating the cause.

White finger (also known as "dead finger" or Raynaud's phenomenon) is associated with vibrating tools. What happens is that the blood vessels in the hand become damaged and eventually spasmodic because of the vibration. When that happens, the skin and muscle tissues can't get enough oxygen and die.

Symptoms include loss of feeling and control in the hands and fingers, numbness and a tingling sensation, blanching of the skin, and a reduced sense of heat, cold and pain. Exposure to cold often brings on the symptoms, or makes them worse. Some workers may become so afflicted they have to wear gloves all the time.

Unfortunately, there is no simple, effective treatment for white finger. However, the condition may improve if the exposure to vibration is removed and the workers are young and healthy enough. Severe cases may require a change in jobs.

Remember: doing any of these motions or activities once or twice for short periods may not seem hazardous. But if they are performed repeatedly over long periods, you are risking hand and wrist trouble that can be both painful and disabling.

Vibration Syndrome

Numbness, pain and whitening of the fingers can be a sign of vibration syndrome, a condition caused by the use of vibrating handtools. Also known as "white finger" or Raynaud's phenomenon, the condition was first described in 1862 by a French physician, Dr. Maurice Raynaud. But, after more than 120 years, it remains one of the most grossly underreported occupational risks.

Part of the reason for this underreporting by workers is that the symptoms come and go. And they are often present at times and under conditions not generally associated with a visit to the doctor's office—early in the morning, or when the hands are wet or cold.

Many physicians and other health professionals underreport vibration syndrome because the whitening effect and loss of feeling also can be signs of other medical conditions. The same symptoms might be the result of such things as fractures, lacerations, connective tissue diseases, vascular disorders such as Buerger's disease, generalized atherosclerosis, or a long history of high blood pressure, among other things.

As recently as 1979, the Bureau of Labor Statistics' Supplementary Data System showed fewer than 40 cases that might have been vibration syndrome. This raised an interesting question: With an estimated 1.5 million workers exposed on the job to hand-arm vibration, was white finger a rare disease, or was there a lot more of it in the workplace that had not been uncovered because of underreporting?

To resolve this question, the National Institute for Occupational Safety and Health (NIOSH) recently completed a comprehensive study of 385 workers at two foundries and a shipyard who used pneumatic chipping hammers and grinders. A similar group, working at the same locations, but without being exposed to vibrating handtools, was used as a control group to measure any differences.

The results of the study showed that 47 percent of the exposed workers in the foundries and 19 percent of the exposed workers in the shipyard had advanced vibration syndrome. Although no workers in the control group were found to have the syndrome, 83 percent of the exposed foundry workers and 64 percent of the exposed shipyard workers had noticeable, but less severe, symptoms.

In order to pinpoint vibration alone as the possible cause, no workers were included in the study who had medical conditions which might have duplicated the symptoms of Raynaud's phenomenon.

The NIOSH study also showed that length of exposure was directly related to the severity of the condition. Signs of varying severity showed up in 31 percent of the foundry workers exposed for 18 months or less; 41 percent exposed from a year and a half to three years, and 71 percent of workers who had been exposed to vibrating handtools for longer than three years. Similar relationships were found among the shipyard workers.

Temporary tingling or numbness in the fingers during or soon after using vibrating handtools is NOT considered vibration syndrome. To be diagnosed as vibration syndrome, the symptoms must be more persistent and come on without provocation, such as immediate exposure to the vibration. In true cases the symptoms usually appear suddenly and are usually brought on by cold. If the exposure continues long enough, the signs and symptoms become more severe and the condition can become irreversible. Workers should see a physician promptly if they experience prolonged symptoms of tingling, numbness or blanched or blue fingers.

Based on its study, NIOSH recommends several steps that could be taken to help reduce exposure to vibrating handtools and to help identify vibration syndrome in its early stages among workers likely to be at risk. These steps include engineering controls (including tool design), medical surveillance, work practices and personal protective equipment.

- All vibrating handtools should be carefully maintained according to the manufacturers' specifications.
- A 10-minute break after each hour of continuous exposure to vibrating handtools may help to reduce the severity of vibration syndrome. However, more research is needed to determine whether other scheduling of rest breaks is more appropriate.
- Workers should wear adequate clothing, especially dry gloves, to keep the body temperature normal and stable. Lowered body temperature can reduce the flow of blood to the extremities and possibly trigger an attack of vibration syndrome.
- Let the tool do the work. Use as light a grip as possible while working safely and maintaining control.

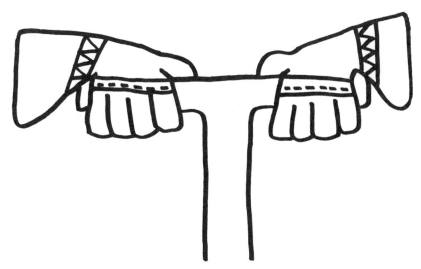

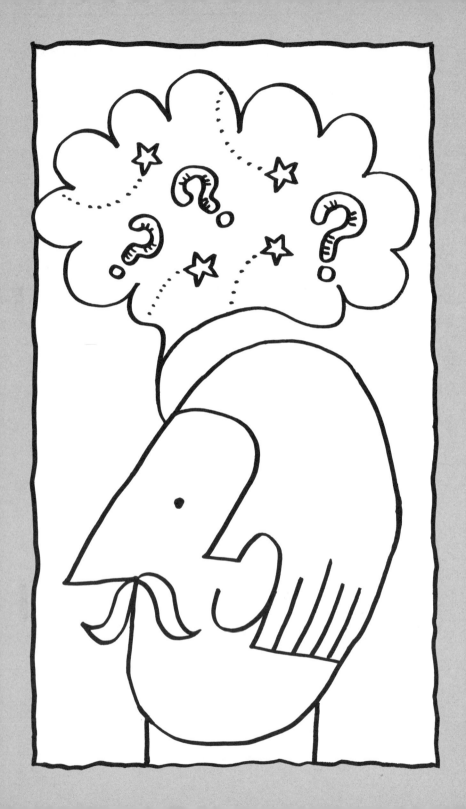

4 Occupational Stress

Can You Worry Yourself Sick?

"I'm worried sick about my job," Sylvia said to her friend as they clocked out.

"For crying out loud," Lonnie chided her. "Snap out of it, will ya? It's all in your head!"

Can you worry yourself sick? Or, are those symptoms you complain about all in your head—psychosomatic, to give them a medical name? The answer to both questions is "yes." You *can* make yourself sick, and it may *begin* in your head.

Psychosomatic is a combination of "psyche" (mind) and "soma" (body). How the two work together to produce psychosomatic conditions is becoming clearer as we learn more about the chemistry of the brain and the body's hormonal system.

Brain chemicals, produced by tiny glands, are what make us react to danger. We jump out of the way of a crazy motorist under the same mental-chemical impulse that prodded a caveman to dodge a saber-tooth tiger.

Let's say your brain senses a threat. The hypothalamus, a small gland deep in the brain, alerts the pituitary gland to release a hormone. That action triggers the adrenal glands to pump out other hormones, including adrenaline. This rush of "high-test" fuel gives us the momentary speed and strength to get out of danger.

So far, so good. The trouble arises when the engine is revved up and kept in high gear for too long, too often, for no good reason. Just as an overworked engine can eventually break down, so can the heart, lungs, blood vessels and stomach lining wear out.

However—and it's important to understand this—the brain itself doesn't make you sick. The trouble probably was already there. Those persistent chemical responses to danger signals from the brain can aggravate existing symptoms or weaknesses already within you. Sylvia's headache, dizziness, or whatever symptoms made her feel "worried sick" very likely could be traced to some physical problem to begin with: high blood pressure, poor circulation, low blood sugar or something else.

103

High blood pressure (hypertension) is often aggravated by emotional stress, although it is not caused by anxiety. The danger for millions of Americans with high blood pressure is that there are no symptoms in about 90 percent of the cases. But under the mind-body responses to stress, the blood pressure can rise and body hormones are secreted at higher levels. These changes can bring on heart disease, kidney damage or other serious complications.

Excessive chemical levels in the brain, brought on by stress and anxiety, are being investigated as potential causes of cancer. Researchers are trying to find a possible link between cancer and the body's immune system, which can be affected by body chemistry.

So, psychosomatic illness is real. It is no longer associated with "goldbricking" or faking a sickness to get out of doing something you don't want to do. It's real. And you are sick. But work with your doctor to find the underlying causes.

Fortunately, the psychosomatic system seems to work the other way, too. If you can "worry yourself sick," shouldn't you be able to "not-worry" yourself into a state of healthy well-being? That intriguing question is being looked into. The results aren't all in, but there is some evidence to suggest that happier people are healthier people.

There are some things you can do yourself to try to reduce the worry and stress in your life. It may not be easy, but try to:

- Identify your fears and worries (not just some nameless dread), and try to think of positive ways to cope with them;
- Balance all the demands of your life without zeroing in on just one of them;
- Set aside regular times for diversions, outside interests, rest and relaxation;
- Don't lean on alcohol or drugs to cure your anxiety; you may wind up with something else to worry about;
- Learn to laugh more; laughter is one of the best tension-breakers you have going for you.

How to Reduce Job Stress

Unlike cancer, lung disease or heart ailments, stress is not a disease in itself. Researchers disagree about whether stress actually can make a person sick. But a fair amount of evidence suggests that stress does impair health and cause mental strain. Several studies have shown that people in stressful jobs have faster heart rates, higher blood pressures, higher cholesterol levels and a greater tendency to smoke heavily. All of these factors can contribute to heart disease.

At least one research team has found the incidence of heart attacks is greater among persons in high stress jobs than it is among workers in low stress occupations. High blood pressure among air traffic controllers was found to be four times as prevalent as among people in less stressful work. Peptic ulcers were twice as prevalent in the same group.

The controllers also had a higher incidence of diabetes, although the connection with the job was not as clearcut as it was for high blood pressure and ulcers. However, diabetes often develops after periods of stress, hard work and frustration.

Other workers who face frequent life and death decisions, like air traffic controllers, are likely to suffer from job stress. These include health care personnel, police officers, pilots, dispatchers and others responsible for public safety.

High-level executive decisions are stressful. So are the tasks of an assembly line worker whose movements are determined by the speed of machinery beyond his or her control. Deadlines create stress for reporters, editors, accountants and others who must work under daily or seasonal time pressures.

The human body responds to stress physically in a predictable way. First, there is a lowering of resistance to infectious disease. Second, the body gears up its defense mechanisms and prepares to act. Adrenaline is released. The heart rate speeds up. Blood pressure rises. Digestive secretions increase.

If this state of readiness is prolonged, scientists believe it can lead to chronic illnesses—cardiovascular disease, ulcers, kidney ailments and perhaps even allergies, arthritis and rheumatism—all caused by the body's repeated attempts to adapt to stress.

In addition, there is another undesirable product—mental strain. The psychological discomfort of stress can be just as disabling as any physical illness. At the very least, the quality of life is impaired. A worker under constant stress is certainly not as happy as he or she might otherwise be.

Unlike chemicals and gases, stress cannot be tasted, smelled or seen. Different people react to stress in different ways. For example, the hard-driving success-oriented person may cope more handily with stress than a less aggressive worker. (Of course, the hard-driving type is also more likely to develop high cholesterol, high blood pressure and, consequently, heart disease.)

Even in similar job situations, different individuals may react differently. One may see the workload as his or her own psychological poison, while another may feel pressured between two supervisors who seem to be making conflicting demands. And, unlike treatments for various specific illnesses, there is no drug or surgery that can be prescribed for a worker troubled by stress. There is only one cure: Remove the source of the stress.

Researchers at the University of Michigan Institute for Social Research have studied job stress for about 20 years. They offer some specific suggestions for reducing stress on the job:

- Train workers to do their jobs as efficiently as possible, using shortcuts wherever possible;
- Rotate people in high stress jobs that cannot be restructured;
- Make sure each person understands his or her responsibilities;
- Distribute work according to workers' capabilities and give some people the right to delegate more work;
- Set up clear lines of communication between workers and supervisors, and reduce the levels of hierarchy within the organization;
- Give employees a voice in decisions that are rightly theirs to make.

Mental Illness in the Workplace

Running through the rich folklore of medicine are various illnesses and diseases that people were too ashamed or frightened to talk about frankly: cancer, tuberculosis, syphilis, gonorrhea. They all fell into that unspeakable category until fairly recently, hiding behind supposedly less harsh names such as "felon," "consumption," and "social disease."

Fortunately, most of us have outgrown this squeamishness and can now discuss—and treat—these illnesses openly and honestly. Unfortunately, there is still an illness that a lot of people seem reluctant to face squarely in themselves, in their families, or among friends. That is mental illness. Yet, at some time in their lives, between 10 and 15 percent of the workers in America will undergo treatment for mental illness. Considerably more will need help.

Let's put this illness in perspective . . . come to grips with the reality of it. To do that, we need to abandon the mistaken notion that "if you don't talk about it, it will go away." It won't.

Mental illness can range from a "nervous breakdown," which may require a long absence from work for treatment, to mildly irrational behavior ("he blew his top") or psychosomatic illness ("my stomach feels like it's tied in knots"). Job stress is a likely villain in most of these cases. In any event, the experience is painful to the individual, the family and friends, and costly in absenteeism and reduced productivity.

Happily, in most cases, the illness will be temporary, the employee will recover, and can look forward to returning to a useful role in his or her organization.

Some companies are beginning to look for the causes of job-related mental illnesses and, when they are identified, taking steps to eliminate them. Any management or union seriously concerned about the welfare of workers must be willing to ask hard questions in the search for causes and prevention of mental illness. For example: Are workers getting the recognition they deserve? Does the company break up established teams, creating insecurity among workers?

There are other factors that can cause stress: the shift system, the pace of production, the amount of control an operator has over the job pace, the pressures of making fast and accurate decisions, the opportunity (or lack of it) for personal interchange. Often there are telltale signs of possible problem areas: departments with high turnover of key personnel, lack of opportunities for relaxation, a breakdown in communications that can leave employees in the dark about any help that is available.

Individuals who may be getting near the end of their rope may show a sudden change in behavior or work patterns. They may take excessive time off for medical reasons, often for vague complaints they can't quite put their fingers on. They may have trouble getting along with coworkers. Their moods may swing widely and quickly between Sunny Jim and Mopey Joe (or Jane).

Curiously, a crackup may not happen while the pressure is on, but in the weeks after it is off. "That's when most people have their breakdowns," says Dr. Gavin Tennent, a British physician and stress authority.

Of equal importance in identifying a worker with a psychological problem is the matter of how to give a fair shake to that individual when he or she returns to work. It takes planning, tact, and a lot of sympathy.

As soon as possible, the returning worker needs to take on responsibilities. If the supervisor or shop steward believes the old job may still be too stressful, reduced responsibilities can be increased gradually in step with the worker's demonstrated ability to cope. If the return is on probation, it should be made clear that this is for a specific time. The worker shouldn't feel that he is under endless scrutiny and that his ability is in doubt. He has enough doubts of his own at this point.

The returning worker also needs to remember what it was like before. Was it quarrelsome, erratic behavior that tipped the scales in the first place? He (or she) probably has used up a lot of credits among supervisors, shop stewards and fellow workers. There are some "dues" to pay in return for the welcome-back vote of confidence.

Remember: It may have taken a long time for the pieces to fall apart. It probably will take time and understanding to put them all back together again. But it is worth repeating: In most cases, the illness will be temporary. The worker will recover. And he or she will be capable once again of fulfilling a useful function.

Workplace Change & 'Technostress'

"What you don't know won't hurt you."—True? Don't bet on it! Like a lot of old sayings, this one makes just as much sense turned upside down and inside out: "What you don't know may, indeed, hurt you." The unknown—the new, the untried, the different—may not hurt you physically, but the fear of it may be painfully uncomfortable.

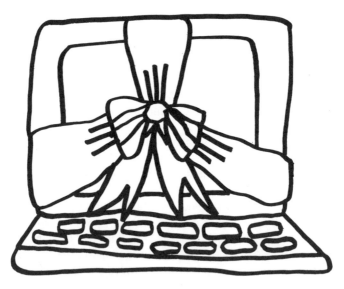

Let's take the case of Gloria, a secretary in a large office. One day her typewriter is replaced with a microcomputer. Gloria has been instructed in its use, but it's still a strange and unknown element in her old work situation, vaguely threatening. She's both excited by the new machine and awed by it. Little telltale signals begin to appear: increased heart rate, rapid breathing, sweaty palms, muscle tension.

Gloria is experiencing "technostress"—the inability, generally temporary, to adapt to the introduction and operation of new technology. This kind of stress affects different people in different ways. Some workers thrive on the challenge of mastering the unknown; others cringe from it.

Some workers will take to a new microcomputer—or any kind of technical innovation—like a duck takes to water, quickly excelling in using it. Often just as quickly, however, the fast learners may become bored. They start experimenting with shortcuts, or putting in information on their own. Errors begin to crop up and stress mounts.

Other employees may just as quickly experience overload trying to learn how to use the new machine while keeping up with the old workload. They may begin to doubt their ability to master the job, or become jealous of those around them who seem to be making faster progress. They may fall back on old work habits to keep up and, when the computer balks, peevishly blame the machine.

There's a fine line between exhilaration and stress. If you're keyed up too tightly for too long, excitement may slip over into stress. Eagerness can become anxiety. Your outlook and behavior may change. Your body may react in a variety of ways—from headache, to stomach cramps, to a nasty disposition, to name just a few.

Craig Brod, author of a recently published book entitled *Technostress,* points out that new technology "changes the nature of work."

Work becomes "machine-dependent." You may feel that you are serving the machine, rather than the other way around. A computer, for example, has its own response time. During the day it may have peaks and valleys. A job that takes 30 minutes at 7 o'clock in the morning may take three times as long by mid-afternoon. That can be frustrating.

Work becomes "information-intensive." The machine may have a voracious appetite for information. And you've got to feed it fast with a "diet" of strange new symbols instead of the everyday language you're used to.

Much of the new technology requires a high degree of teamwork. Whole units of people, not just individuals, have to mesh smoothly through the organization. This may require rethinking old methods. The old top-to-bottom flow of information may need a close look from managers and supervisors. Concentration on individual effort may have to be restudied, by employees and management alike, with an eye toward improving group productivity.

Technostress can be managed. Learn all you can about the technology. Find out how your job fits into the whole operation. Learn at firsthand—not by hearsay—what to expect and how you can deal with it. Practice coping skills; think "I can," not "I can't."

Another old saying—"Familiarity breeds contempt"—may not be true, either, in this case. Familiarity with the new technology may breed respect, both for your machine and for yourself in adapting to its use. That could raise your comfort level at work, as well as your productivity.

Reducing Heart Attack Risks

Heart attacks take the lives of more than 670,000 people in the United States each year—one and a half times as many as battle deaths claimed in all the wars Americans fought in so far this century. Many thousands of these victims are in the prime of their lives—men and women who had "never been sick a day in their lives."

What does medical science know about this killer?

What can you do to reduce your chances of heart attack?

First, by studying the medical records and living habits of thousands of middle-age people, scientists have been able to pinpoint certain risk factors that were present in those who had heart attacks.

This identification of the major risks is one of the most encouraging advances in recent medical knowledge. It tells us the precautions all of us can take to increase our chances of living longer and enjoying good health.

Second, in answer to the second question, here's what the American Heart Association says: "With the advice of a doctor, most people can regulate the habits and physical conditions that may be endangering their hearts."

Here are the risk factors. It appears that any one of them increases the risk of a heart attack. Two or more multiplies that risk.

- High blood pressure
- High levels of cholesterol or other fatty substances in the blood
- Excess weight
- Diabetes
- Lack of exercise
- Cigarette smoking
- A family history of heart attacks in middle age

Do one or more of those warning signs hit home? Don't panic. Working with your doctor, there are things you can do to reduce the risks—even in the case of heredity, over which it might seem you have no control.

The fact that a close relative died between the ages of 40 and 60 from the complications of atherosclerosis could mean that a tendency to the disease runs in your family. However, you may or may not inherit the tendency. And, even if you do inherit the tendency, it is not inevitable that you will have the disease.

If the heredity thing bothers you, turn it to your advantage. You have been given an early warning that other people might not receive. You can take steps to reduce the known risks. For instance: Although the cause of the most common type of hypertension (high blood pressure) is unknown, it's a controllable disease. Drugs can lower the pressure. A sensible diet can bring the weight down. You can cut out smoking cigarettes, and modify living habits that are causing stress.

Even when times are tough, most Americans enjoy a standard of living that is higher than is found in other parts of the world. Ironically, our health often suffers because of it.

We tend to eat a lot of meat and dairy products—foods that are high in saturated fats. We eat a lot of eggs and some organ meats (all of which are high in cholesterol) as well as high-calorie foods. A diet rich in these types of foods tends to raise the level of cholesterol and fatty substances in the blood. And these blood levels of fats, in turn, contribute to the development of atherosclerosis which raises the risk of a heart attack.

It would be impossible—and understandable—to cut out all saturated fats in the diet. There are some in foods you need. The goal is to raise the proportion of polyunsaturated fats to saturated fats. Many people do this by eating more fish and poultry instead of meat, using skimmed (fat-free) or low-fat milk, and cooking with vegetable oils instead of butter or lard.

As for smoking cigarettes—DON'T!

Will it help to quit now even though you've been a heavy smoker for years? You bet! Studies show that people who gave up smoking have a lower death rate from heart attack than people who kept on smoking. After a period of years, the death rate for those who stopped was nearly as low as that of people who never smoked. Some abnormally changed lung tissue gradually reverts to normal after smoking is eliminated.

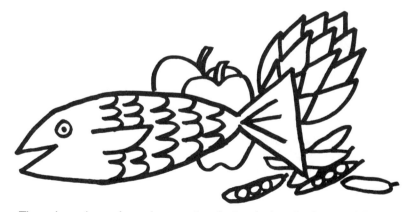

There is no brass-bound guarantee that reducing the known risks will prevent heart attacks. But most of the scientific evidence today points that way.

High Blood Pressure

High blood pressure, or hypertension, is a chronic condition in which blood is pumped through the body at higher than normal pressure. According to the American Heart Association, nearly 34 million American adults have high blood pressure, a major contributing factor in heart attacks. Even more adults show blood pressures in the borderline range.

The condition is treacherous because it has no characteristic symptoms. A victim can have the disease for years and not know it. If uncontrolled, high blood pressure also can kill by seriously damaging vital organs such as the kidneys, as well as through cardiovascular damage.

Generally, anything that decreases the size of the arteries can contribute to high blood pressure. The heart—like any other pump—has to exert greater pressure to propel a given amount of blood through a narrower opening than it would if the passage were larger. Studies have shown that a number of factors can contribute to this narrowing of the arteries. These include cigarette smoking, stress, excessive noise, or the deposits of plaques on the inside walls of the arteries, often caused by too much cholesterol in the diet.

Fortunately, a change in lifestyle, plus the use of prescribed drugs, can often control high blood pressure. However, they cannot cure it. Medication also can control congestive heart failure by helping the heart muscle function more normally, and by ridding the body of excess fluids that have built up in the lungs and other organs.

Unfortunately, medical science at this time doesn't know a lot about what causes high blood pressure. Between 90 and 95 percent of the time, the diagnosis is simply "essential hypertension," or high blood pressure from unknown causes.

In order to measure blood pressure, medical science had to find some precise pressure measurement outside the body, and then relate that known pressure to the amount of pressure the heart was using to pump blood through the arteries. A column of mercury was selected because it takes a specific amount of pressure to raise a column of mercury a specific height, measured in millimeters. The higher the pressure, the higher the column is raised. This is a purely arbitrary device, but it provides reference points, or a framework, for setting the boundaries for "normal" blood pressure. Here's how it works:

The doctor, nurse or other health professional will wrap a cuff around your upper arm and squeeze a bulb which inflates a balloon-like inner lining. This builds up a pressure which eventually collapses an artery underneath. A stethoscope is placed over an exposed spot on the collapsed artery, usually where your elbow bends. Then the air is gradually let out. When the pressure in the tight cuff falls below the pressure in the artery, the stethoscope picks up the sound of the first spurt of blood. This point on the millimeter scale is recorded as the highest component of your blood pressure—the systolic.

More air is let out until the cuff no longer restricts the flow of blood and there is no sound of turbulence. The point where the sound disappears is the lowest component of blood pressure—the diastolic.

Systolic refers to the rhythmic contraction of the heart, especially the ventricles, or valves, by which blood is driven through the aorta or pulmonary. Diastolic refers to the rhythmic relaxation and dilation of the heart cavities during which the cavities are filled with blood, ready for the next go around—over and over for as long as you live.

Clench your fist and alternately squeeze and relax, squeeze and relax, and you will get a rough idea of this constant outflow and inflow functioning of the heart pump.

Normal blood pressure has been set arbitrarily as lower than 140 systolic and 90 diastolic. Those numbers were picked after investigations of many groups of people over long periods of time showed that's where most of the blood pressures happened to be. Pressure between 140 and 159 systolic and 90 and 94 diastolic is considered borderline high blood pressure. Anything higher than these sets of numbers is high blood pressure.

High blood pressure, or hypertension, must be diagnosed and treated by a physician. Numerous studies have established a definite connection between the condition and various cardiovascular ailments such as heart attacks and strokes.

But despite its stealthy and deadly nature, there is a positive side to this story of the silent killer. High blood pressure can, in most cases, be controlled by prescribed medication, faithfully used by the patient. Re-

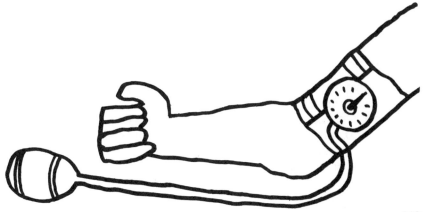

member, too, that the patient also has control. Altering one's lifestyle to a less hectic pace can be helpful. By following a prescribed diet, a sufferer from high blood pressure may regulate the level of cholesterol in the body.

And a final reminder: Cigarette smokers clearly have a higher rate of heart attacks and strokes than nonsmokers. If you decide to stop smoking, you can be reassured by studies showing that the death rate from cardiovascular disease can drop nearly as low as for those who have never smoked. You have a choice.

What Is a Stroke?

What we commonly call a "stroke" is an accident that happens to an artery supplying blood to the brain. About half a million Americans suffer strokes each year, 4 out of 10 of whom die as a result, making stroke the No. 3 killer right after heart disease and cancer.

Strokes most often occur in older people, with the peak age period beginning in the 60s, although they may occur before middle age. Nearly twice as many men suffer strokes as women.

Grave as these statistics are, however, there is a brighter side. Of the estimated 2 million stroke victims alive today, about 30 percent have returned to work or to their normal activities, according to the National Institute of Neurological and Communicative Disorders and Stroke (NINCDS).

Another 55 percent of these stroke survivors are disabled but still can carry on such daily activities of life as dressing themselves, eating and so on. And promising strides are being made in preventive medicine and rehabilitative techniques that could make the future even brighter for stroke victims.

What is a stroke? This "cerebrovascular accident," to give it the medical name, can be the result of any one of the following:

1. A clot (thrombus) forms in a narrowed part of a major artery to the brain, thus slowing the blood flow. This is the cerebral thrombosis you hear about. It is the commonest cause of a stroke. It frequently happens to people who have arteriosclerosis (hardening of the arteries), often associated with high blood pressure.

2. An "embolism" (blockage) forms in a blood vessel in some other part of the body. This can be caused by a clot, gas bubbles, clumps of bacteria or droplets of fat. The plug, instead of remaining stationary, is

swept along by the blood stream until it lodges in one of the arteries that supplies the brain. This wandering clot is called an embolus.
3. A weakened spot in the walls of an artery balloons out under pressure and leaks or bursts. The cerebral hemorrhage floods into the brain, damaging or destroying the surrounding tissue.

Some people identify a stroke with the aftermath of the accident—the effects of the interference with the brain's blood supply—instead of the primary cause, the accident itself. These aftereffects can take a number of forms: paralysis, loss of speech, inability to remember, visual impairment and so on.

The reason the disability can take so many different forms is that various areas of the brain are responsible for directing, by way of the nerves, all the body's different functions. Depending on which message center in the brain is put out of commission by lack of its nourishing blood, the area it controls will be affected by the stroke.

Our bodies are "wired" in a crisscross pattern of nerves. An injury to the left side of the brain will affect the body's right side functions, and vice versa.

The very word "stroke" reminds some people of a lightning strike—a bolt out of the blue. But strokes often give a warning. We call this warning TIA. That stands for the medical term "transient ischemic attack." Transient means the attack comes and goes. Ischemic means lack of sufficient blood. These fleeting attacks—often called mini-strokes—result from a momentary reduction in the flow of blood through a narrowed artery.

Mini-stroke symptoms include numbness or weakness of an arm, leg or side of the face; dizziness, a tingling ("pins and needles") sensation, slurred speech or impaired vision in one eye. Although these signs could be due to other conditions, you should consider them warnings to see your doctor promptly. Some experts in the field report that as many as half of the people who subsequently suffered strokes had also experienced a TIA beforehand.

Recovery from a stroke depends on how much of the brain has been permanently damaged. Sometimes a control center of the brain will not be totally wiped out and patients may be able, with therapy, to relearn a skill. Other areas of the brain, not affected by the stroke, can also be taught to take over some of the jobs previously performed by the damaged areas.

Rehabilitation from a stroke is a team effort in which the family, the patient, the family doctor and many experts—from dietitians to physical therapists to psychologists—can play key roles. Above all, the patient's "will to win" can spell the difference between success and failure.

Alcoholism

If you work in a factory or office with 100 other employees, chances are that about six of your fellow workers may be drinking on the job. They aren't celebrating a promotion or some red-letter day in their lives. They simply can't get through the day—any day—without a certain level of alcohol in their bloodstreams.

They are part of the army of 6.5 million men and women categorized as employed alcoholics by the National Institute of Alcohol Abuse and Alcoholism (NIAAA). The total number of alcoholics in this country, both in and out of the labor force, is estimated at 10 million by the National Council on Alcoholism (NCA) out of a total of 100 million Americans who drink alcoholic beverages.

One in every four is a white collar worker. Nearly one-third—30 percent—are blue collar workers. The other 45 percent are professionals or managers. Most of them are between the ages of 35 and 50. Among them are individuals of all races, religions, economic and social standings. An increasing number are women.

Alcoholism was recognized as a disease in 1956 by the American Medical Association. Despite the findings of medical science in recent years, however, alcoholism is rated as the nations's most untreated, treatable illness by the National Council on Alcoholism. It ranks third behind cancer and heart disease in total fatalities, according to the NCA.

Because so many cases of alcoholism go undetected and untreated among the nation's workers, the disease contributes to the $15 billion chalked up to lost production every year, according to the NIAAA.

Excessive absenteeism is probably one of the most visible symptoms of the working alcoholic. Statistics show that the alcoholic misses an

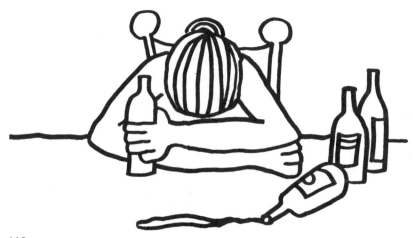

average of 22 days a year, most frequently on Mondays and Fridays. Even worse is on-the-job absenteeism. The alcoholic may be at his or her regular work station, but suffering from a hangover, loss of memory, impaired muscle control, or altered judgment that can have serious effects on job performance.

A number of standards have been set up by which we can measure the difference between social or recreational drinking and alcoholism. For example, whenever an individual's drinking interferes with his health, job, family or social relationships—and he continues to drink—that is alcoholism. There is no real difference between heavy or problem drinking and alcoholism. Heavy drinking is early alcoholism.

Why a person drinks is another indicator. A drinker may drink—away from the job—for reasons of conviviality, relaxation or simply because he or she likes the taste of a particular concoction. The alcoholic, on the other hand, uses alcohol in ever-increasing amounts as a crutch to help him cope with normal, everyday stress.

Alcohol produces two seemingly contradictory effects on the body. It acts both as a sedative and an irritant on the central nervous system. When an alcoholic uses liquor to relieve stress, the initial sedative effect, for a limited time, overcomes the irritant factor. But when the sedative effect wears off, the individual must consume more to overcome the irritating factors. In time, more and more alcohol is required to achieve the desired level of relief from stress. And this sets up a vicious cycle. More alcohol leads to more stress which leads to more alcohol.

Recovery is a process of breaking this cycle. Perhaps the best-known treatment program is that offered through Alcoholics Anonymous. AA was founded in the 1930s by two alcoholics and has grown to a worldwide organization with a membership in excess of 1 million. After expressing an honest desire to stop drinking, the alcoholic finds in AA a supportive interaction program with other recovering alcoholics. Some alcoholics may need additional counseling and therapy from professional sources.

In some cases, it may be necessary for the alcoholic to begin a program of recovery under medical supervision, starting with detoxification. This can take about a week in a hospital, followed by as much as a month of treatment for related health problems, such as malnutrition.

Because of its tremendous economic cost, employee alcoholism is treated more and more in industry by in-house recovery programs.

While the alcoholic worker remains a major problem for industry and business, with devastating consequences for individuals and families, the outlook is not all bleak. Recovery rates of 65 to 80 percent among alcoholics enrolled in treatment programs are indicated by figures from the National Council on Alcoholism.

Drug Abuse

Drug abuse among American workers is much like the scary noise outside a camper's tent at night: Uneasily, we know there's something out there, but we don't know exactly how big or menacing it is.

We do have some clues about the widespread and growing problem of drug abuse among the general population. They are not reassuring. And, since the workforce cuts across all racial, cultural, social and economic lines, we can be reasonably certain that the national problem is showing up in the mills and mines, the factories, offices and shops of America.

One study, by the National Institute of Drug Abuse (NIDA) in 1974, placed the number of workers abusing drugs at 6 million. A more recent study indicates that figure may be conservative.

In a retrospective study spanning the years 1962-1980, NIDA found that 68 percent of the 18-to-25-year-old age group had used marijuana in 1980 compared to only 4 percent for the same age group 18 years earlier. The number who had tried cocaine, heroin, hallucinogens, or inhalants had risen to 33 percent for 1980 compared to 3 percent in the first year covered by the survey.

Another study called the National Survey of Drug Abuse, commissioned by NIDA, threw more distressing light on the subject. A total of 7,000 Americans 12 years of age and older were questioned about their non-medical use of drugs between 1972 and 1979. The respondents were classified as Youth (12-17), Young Adults (18-25), and Older Adults (over 25).

That survey found that among youths and older adults, experience with marijuana and cocaine had doubled in that seven-year period. The percentage of cocaine use among young adults tripled. Marijuana use increased from 48 to 68 percent.

Federal Strategy, compiled and updated periodically by the President's domestic policy staff, in its 1979 issue gave the following numbers of people using selected legal and illegal drugs for non-medical purposes in 1977:

- Marijuana, 16,210,000
- Amphetamines, 1,780,000
- Cocaine, 1,640,000
- Tranquilizers, 1,360,000
- Hallucinogens, 1,140,000
- Barbituates, 1,060,000
- Heroin, 550,000

Given the across-the-board makeup of the American workforce, this means that there are a lot of people out there punching in every day who are in no shape to work or are not showing up at all. The results for workers, business and industry are excessive absenteeism, higher accident risks and poor job performance.

Despite the mounting evidence of widespread and growing drug abuse throughout society, industry has been slow to respond to the problem. Reliable estimates indicate there are probably no more than 600 employee assistance programs in operation which have an effective drug abuse component.

Part of the reluctance to tackle the drug problem is a mistaken belief that, if a company had such a program, it would reflect adversely on the caliber of their personnel. Other employers simply don't know about the variety of treatment programs available or how effective they can be. Still others—like the camper who simply hides under the cover and pretends the noise is a twig snapping—say that, to their knowledge, there is no drug problem and no need for a treatment program.

In contrast are the company drug programs that are working effectively, often in conjunction with similar assistance for alcoholics. The National Association on Drug Abuse Problems (NADAP), with headquarters in New York City, assists some 75 companies throughout the country in setting up and maintaining drug abuse programs. NADAP's advice: Make distinctions between the weekend recreational users, the self-medicating person who takes a substance in a regular fashion in a limited quantity for a specific purpose, and finally, the intensive user for whom life centers around drugs.

The record shows that the greatest success in getting users off drugs

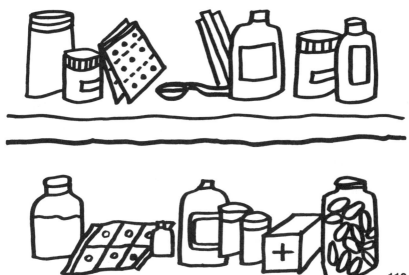

has been through companies and unions that have made drug abuse services an integral part of their overall medical programs.

Drug abuse is a real and growing problem, both for individual workers, unions and industry as a whole. That's reality—not a scary possibility. But just as real, fortunately, is the fact that kick-the-habit programs can work.

Compulsive Gambling

Compulsive gambling is an illness, recognized as such by both the medical and psychiatric professions. This doesn't mean, of course, that everybody who gambles is sick. As with drinking alcohol, there are varying degrees of gambling. Millions of people enjoy going to the racetrack, or attending weekly bingo parties, or having a few of the guys—and everything that will be said here also applies to women—in for a regular Friday night poker game.

These casual gamblers—even the habitual ones—use gambling as a means of socializing, loosening up to relieve tension and stress, feeling the glow of satisfaction that follows a big win. They also know there's a chance of losing. And when they've had enough excitement, or when the losses become too heavy, they break it off and move on to other activities.

The compulsive gambler, on the other hand (like his counterpart, the compulsive drinker) doesn't know when to quit. Or, to be more accurate, can't quit. Control has been lost. The gambler is in the grip of an addiction, an obsessive urge the victim simply can't deny. Jobs suffer. Families suffer. The person's health can go to pieces. The inevitable downward spiral points to social, economic, and emotional collapse, including—in many cases—attempted suicide.

How many of these unfortunates are there? No one knows for sure. Estimates range from a couple of million to as high as 10 million. The few studies that have been made say they range in age from 16 to 70, with the majority between the ages of 20 and 50. Men greatly outnumber women by anywhere from 5 to 1 to 20 to 1. They can be found in all economic and social classes.

Why do they do it? Psychiatrists and psychologists have been trying to answer that question since the early 1900s. They have offered numerous possible explanations.

Robert L. Custer, M.D., a national authority on gambling, wrote a few years ago: ". . . the compulsive gambler gambles to escape or avoid reality, doing this in a manner which creates a fantasy world in which one can feel important, challenged, powerful, influential, or respected. The need for these feelings likely reflects the very areas in which the gambler feels inadequate." Many compulsive gamblers had, or feel they had, a deprived childhood, unnoticed or unloved.

Although recognized as an illness, treatment of compulsive gambling is still relatively in its infancy. The first systematic program was established only 11 years ago by Dr. Custer at the Brecksville Division of the Veterans Administration Medical Center in Ohio.

Noting the great similarity in the personality characteristics of compulsive gamblers and alcoholics, and the remarkable similarity also in the progressive course and development of these disorders, the founders patterned their treatment program along the lines of Alcoholics Anonymous. Several recovery centers are in operation around the country. Some require a stay in a hospital; others operate on an out-patient basis. The Veterans Administration has taken a lead in treatment of compulsive gambling.

Before these professionally staffed centers had been set up, Gamblers Anonymous was founded in 1957. The organization has grown steadily over the years. There are now several hundred GA groups around the world. Like AA, membership is never solicited. The only requirement for membership is an honest desire to stop gambling. Help is only given at the request of the compulsive gambler.

GA members meet regularly, give each other emotional support and practical assistance, and help each other work through the "Twelve Steps"—a series of acknowledgments and resolutions by the compulsive gambler. There are also fellowships for families of the gamblers.

GA groups are listed in the telephone directories of most large cities. In other areas, information can be obtained from state and local departments of human services, or health and welfare, or from family service agencies.

It is not an easy path to follow, but the rewards of success are tremendous—physically, emotionally and financially.

The Mystery of Sleep

Everybody does it, but nobody knows exactly why. Not doing it isn't fatal, so far as anybody knows. But not doing it can produce definite physical results—irritability, lack of concentration. Deprived of it long enough, you might hallucinate—see things that aren't there, hear noises from nowhere. What is this mysterious activity? Sleep.

Sleep (or, most often, the *lack* of it) is a problem for many shift workers. The constant rotation between shifts interferes with the body's "circadian rhythm." This is the "internal clock" we all have inside us that marks the daily ebb and flow pattern of our body functions, including sleeping and waking.

The word "circadian" comes from "circa" and "dia." Put together, they translate roughly into "around day." Left to itself, the human circadian rhythm generally follows a 25-hour day. This "extra" hour—compared with regular clock time—may be especially significant for shift workers.

Taking into account the "overlap" of the internal clock, sleep researchers recently concluded that work schedules that rotate should be arranged so that workers would move forward to the next shift, rather than back to the preceding one. A dramatic drop in complaints about insomnia was recorded in a test of workers at the Great Salt Lake Minerals and Chemicals Corp., Ogden, Utah, when the suggested new shift pattern was put into effect.

The reason this switch seems to help isn't entirely clear. But it suggests that the forward movement of the work schedule may take advantage of the body's circadian rhythm preference for a slightly longer day. You have the momentum of that extra hour to carry you over into the following shift, making adjustment easier than if you moved back.

It is interesting to note that people kept in isolation, deprived of their wristwatches and natural sunlight, nevertheless often continue to operate on a 25-hour cycle—the rising and falling tides of their lives still governed by their internal clocks.

Why the day is split between periods of sleep and wakefulness is not fully understood. We can measure changes in body functions during sleep. The body temperature falls slightly and reaches its lowest point about 4 o'clock in the morning. The blood pressure falls, the rate of

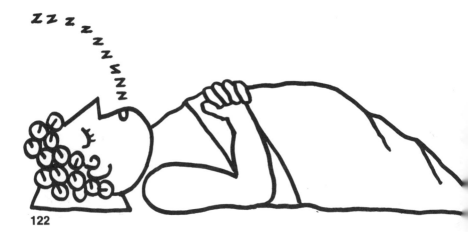

breathing slows, and the pulse rate drops by about 10 percent. The kidneys are less active, and muscle tone slackens.

But the "why" of these physiological processes is poorly understood. One likely reason we sleep is to provide us with a period of growth and the regeneration of body cells. The secretion of the growth hormone somatotropin occurs almost exclusively during sleep.

There is no "required" amount of sleep. In general, most healthy people sleep between five and 10 hours at a stretch, with the majority sleeping for seven or eight hours. However, one thing is sure: People who regularly sleep less than three hours almost invariably complain. And for the majority of "normal" sleepers, a bad night's sleep is usually followed by feelings of tiredness the next day.

Insomnia can be caused by a number of things, plain discomfort being one of the most common. This could be anything from arthritis to a peptic ulcer to lying in a certain position that produces uncomfortable sensation in an arm or leg, particularly if the circulation is poor. Your sleep also can be interfered with if you're worried or depressed, if you're in different surroundings, or if your routine has changed—such as the shift work mentioned earlier.

Whatever the original cause of insomnia, anxiety over loss of sleep often sets up a vicious circle. The more you worry about it, the less likely you are to fall asleep. Insomnia, in itself, is not dangerous, nor does it have any long-term effects. Deprived long enough, people eventually give in to an overwhelming sleepiness.

If insomnia becomes a problem, see your doctor. He may prescribe sleeping pills. Most likely, he'll also look for the underlying cause. If there is a cause—and there usually is—it's better to correct the cause than just to treat the symptom.

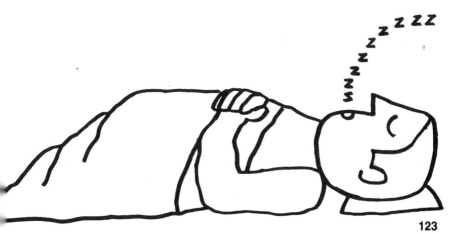

Shiftwork and the Body's 'Clock'

Shiftwork seems to suit some people. Others tolerate it at best or thoroughly dislike it. The main reason for this liking or not liking shiftwork probably is explained by how the individual's biological rhythms are affected. The first group may adjust with little if any difficulty. The others—the majority—may have a number of problems, all of which can affect their health.

All of us—in fact every living thing from plants to insects to humans—have these biological rhythms. This pattern of rising and falling activity is like the rising and falling of the tides. In humans, these changes correspond to the day and night cycle. These 24-hour rhythms are called circadian rhythms, and influence a number of body functions, such as temperature, pulse rate, blood pressure, hormone levels, etc.

In a normal pattern of working by day and sleeping by night, these body functions are at a peak during the day and drop to their lowest point at night. Our "internal clock" is influenced by light and dark and, to a considerable extent, by what everybody else is doing.

Now, let's turn day into night—in a manner of speaking—as shiftwork does for a lot of people. The low point of their biological rhythms, normally a time of rest and reduced activity, now comes at a time of peak work demands. Later, when the shift is over, they have to try to sleep when their activity cycle is on the upswing.

Shiftworkers, especially those on the night shift, on the average get one or two hours less sleep than dayworkers. Not only do they get less sleep, but the quality of the sleep and its ability to refresh the worker is less during the day.

Working shifts also seems to cause more digestive illnesses than work during normal daytime hours, and to aggravate existing ones. Ulcers and constipation are more common among shiftworkers than day workers, according to researchers.

When switching to another shift, some workers may lose their appetites, while others may react by overeating. These changes are often aggravated by irregular meals, poorer food in many cases, and eating when the body's digestive system is at a low point. Fatigue and disruption of the central nervous system, often brought on by lack of sound sleep, also can have adverse effects on digestion.

Several studies indicate that there are more accidents at night, and that they tend to be more severe. The effects of fatigue and disrupted bodily rhythms must share the blame for the higher accident rates on night shifts. Many experts also believe that when the body is out of rhythm and under stress and strain, it is more susceptible to the effects of physical agents (noise, vibration, radiation) and chemical agents (fumes, gases, dusts).

These conditions are made worse if there are inadequate first aid and medical facilities on the night shift—a situation that is not uncommon in some workplaces.

Women have a special physical problem with shiftwork. The altered work pattern not only disrupts the normal 24-hour rhythms; it can disrupt longer rhythms as well, such as the menstrual cycle of about 28 days. Shiftwork can cause the missing of periods, irregular periods and more painful periods.

A number of proper and useful suggestions have been made for responding to these problems faced by shiftworkers. They include:

- A greater say in designing flexible work and shift rosters, and choice of shifts;
- A reduction of workhours on shift, and more breaks;
- First aid and medical facilities kept available;
- Better meal and transportation facilities;
- Medical checkups every six months at management's expense and in paid time.

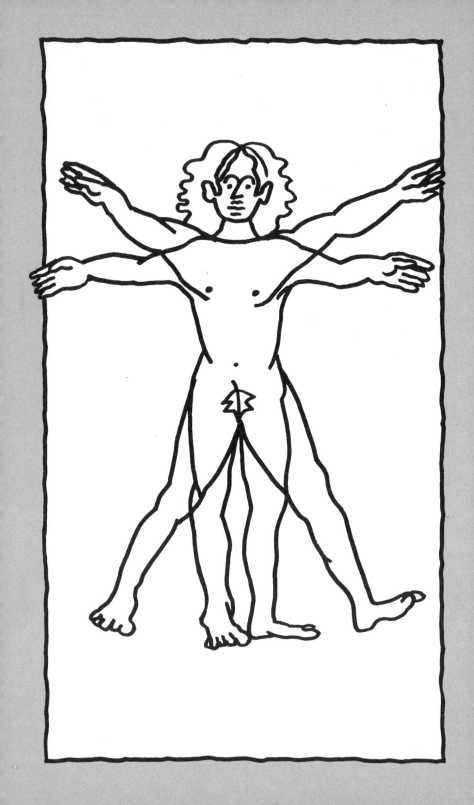

5 Body Systems

Cancer's Terrible Toll

This year, 785,000 people in this country will find out they have cancer. About 405,000 will die of the disease—one every 80 seconds. At the present rate, and it has been going up steadily, one in four Americans now living will eventually have cancer. The disease will strike two of every three families.

In terms of medical treatment and the loss of earnings because of disability and early death, cancer costs the U.S. about $30 billion a year. Yet, in the war on this harrowing and costly epidemic, the nation currently is budgeting only about one-thirtieth of the annual toll in dollars—something over $1 billion. And only 5 to 10 percent of that amount is being allocated to the preventive aspects of cancer.

These grim statistics can be valuable if they prod us to take a clearer look at the need to shift our priorities. They will not serve a good purpose if they cause us to shrug off the dread risk with a fatalistic, head-in-the-sand attitude that "everything causes cancer" and let it go at that.

So, very briefly, what are some of the things we know about cancer—and don't know?

First, just what is cancer? The term describes a variety of different diseases with a number of causes. Basically, in all forms of cancer the body's cell division system goes haywire and this leads to an uncontrolled growth of abnormal cells. A cancer generally starts out in one place and, unless checked, can spread deeper into the affected organ and throughout the body by way of the blood or lymph system. If this spread is extensive enough, the person dies.

What causes cancer? Frankly, there is no simple answer. Scientists have identified a number of possible causes. These include viruses, radiation (produced by X-ray equipment, radioactive elements and even the sun), and chemicals, both natural and manmade, that are found in everything from toxic industrial wastes to food and water.

Experts agree that a number of other factors help to determine whether a person develops cancer and, if so, how quickly it will spread. These factors include heredity, age, lifestyle and general health.

The various causes of cancer are complicated by another factor: we live in a chemical-laden society. It is almost impossible to escape a variety of suspected or proven cancer-causing agents. And studies show that some substances acting together produce more tumors in a shorter time than either one by itself. For example, lung cancer is enormously more frequent among asbestos workers who smoke than in the nonsmoking general population because of this multiplying effect.

What can be done? First, let's look at the roots of the problem. The World Health Organization estimates that between 75 and 85 percent of all cancers are caused by environmental exposure. The everyday environment for most Americans includes the places they work.

Since the great majority of cancers are caused by agents in the environment, it follows that potentially they are preventable. In short, get rid of the substance and you get rid of the risk. But this isn't as simple in practice as it is to say. Costs, differences of opinion among agencies about how best to tackle the problem, the long time delay between exposure and the appearance of cancers—all of these things have contributed to the nation's failure to adequately protect workers and the general public.

There are some things that can be done, however. We need to:

- Tell workers now exposed to cancer-causing agents about their risks, and put controls on such hazardous situations;
- Report the use of such substances to appropriate agencies for enforcement and compliance purposes;
- Locate workers who may have been exposed in the past and channel them into screening programs aimed at early detection;
- Pre-test all new chemicals for any cancer-causing properties, and screen those already in use;
- Set up tumor registries throughout the country, a data source where all cancer cases would be reported so scientists can get one more handle on the magnitude and nature of the problem;
- Establish cancer "hotlines" for public information.

Tips on Occupational Cancer

"I'm a roofer," Harvey said. "Is there any chance of getting cancer from the things I do or the materials I use?"

"Woodworking is an old trade," Nick said. "There can't be any cancer risk in what I do, like the fellows who work with chemicals. Or, is there?"

"A lot of the guys in my shop—we do brake and clutch work—talk about cancer from asbestos," Lonnie said. "Is there anything to that?"

Well, there's good news and bad news.

The good news is that more workers today, like Harvey and Nick and Lonnie, are concerned about occupational cancer. They are learning about how the risks can be reduced. They know how to spot the early warning signs of cancer.

The bad news is that the answer to all three questions at the beginning of this column is, "Yes." There is risk for roofers, woodworkers, anybody who works with or around asbestos, and for many more men and women in other occupations.

There is good reason for workers to be concerned, as well as their families. The American Cancer Society reports that one out of every four Americans contracts some form of cancer during his or her lifetime. And, if you're an average reader, one of those Americans has died since you started reading—about one every 80 seconds!

Here are a few high-risk trades and operations, the particular carcinogens (cancer-causing agents) that workers may be exposed to, and parts of the body most likely to be affected:

Roofing trades. Coal-tar pitch volatiles, asphalt. (Lungs, mouth, larynx, esophagus)
Woodworking. Solvents, chlorinated hydrocarbons, organic dusts. (Nasal membranes)
Automobile clutch and brake maintenance. Asbestos. (Lungs, mesothelium—lining of pulmonary and abdominal cavities)
Asbestos fabrication, insulation. Asbestos. (Same as above)
Uranium mining, processing. Radiation. (Lungs, lymphatic system)
Rubber manufacture. Benzene. (Bone marrow)
Dye industry. Benzidine (Bladder)
Metal working. Chromium, arsenic. (Respiratory system)
Oil refining. Polycyclic hydrocarbons. (White blood cells)
Coke oven work. Coke oven emissions. (Kidneys, lungs)
Plastics production. Vinyl chloride. (Liver)

This is only a partial list. Many more jobs could be added, especially those in which asbestos is a factor. Asbestos is found in practically every industry today in some form or another—either as part of the manufacturing process, or as a part of the plant's insulation. And its use has been increasing steadily over the last 20 years or so.

Another large group of workers may risk skin cancer from excessive exposure to sunlight. These include gardeners, foresters, utility lineworkers, farmers and so on.

The partial list of high-risk occupations is from a booklet called *More Than a Paycheck: An Introduction to Occupational Cancer.* The booklet is put out by the U.S. Department of Labor, Occupational Safety and Health Administration.

Occupational cancer is a problem of staggering proportions, based on all we know today. But what we don't know is even more worrisome. We don't know, for instance, how many cancer-causing agents still un-identified are present in the workplace. Industry begins using a new chemical—often untested—about every 20 minutes. We don't know the effects that may appear many years from now from exposure that is taking place at this moment.

Most experts agree that the only sure way to reduce the threat of occupational cancer is to prevent exposure in the first place. Meanwhile, you can check seven key signals that may mean cancer is present:

- Any unusual bleeding or discharge through the mouth, nose, vagina, anus or bladder.
- A sore or ulcer that doesn't heal normally.
- Indigestion or difficulty in swallowing.
- Much hoarseness or persistent cough.
- Some changes in bowel or bladder habits.
- Hardening or lump in the breast or other part of the body.
- Changes in the color or size of a wart or mole.

None of these signals means for sure that you have cancer. But if any of them lasts for more than two weeks, you should see a doctor. Chances are good that it is *not* cancer, but only a doctor can tell for sure.

Reproductive Hazards

Working women who want to have children can be exposed to reproductive hazards at three critical points—before conception, during pregnancy, and after birth. Fertility, the ability to get pregnant, can be affected by any toxic substance that causes irregular menstruation, changes in the egg, or in the body's hormone system which regulates the woman's reproductive cycle. But beyond this general statement, there is a woeful lack of solid medical data to pinpoint the fertility risks of the workplace.

There is evidence that exposure to polychlorinated biphenyls (PCBs), used in the electronics industry, may cause infertility. Other suspected hazards, about which more study is needed, involve solvents, excessive heat, and radiation.

A number of fairly common substances found in the workplace can cause cancer under certain conditions. Should cancer strike the reproductive organs themselves, this may interfere with conception. The discovery of such a cancer usually leads to the surgical removal of the organ.

Even if the reproductive organs are not involved, cancer in other parts of the body may indirectly affect the reproductive capabilities in other ways. Radiation or chemotherapy used to treat cancer are extremely hazardous to the egg as well as to the developing fetus in pregnant women. Conception is not advisable during such treatment.

Mutations, or changes in the genetic material or body cells, are another cause of pre-conception concern. The hereditary units of living cells are made up of genes. Genes regulate the cells' activity and are combined into strands called chromosomes. This genetic material is the blueprint that determines what characteristics children inherit from their parents.

Most mutations are harmful, although the harm may not be visibly apparent. Sometimes these changes can cause the cells to divide abnormally, resulting in cancer—the unchecked growth and multiplication of cells. The functioning of the cells also may be altered, as happens in sickle cell anemia.

From conception until birth, the fetus is particularly vulnerable to toxic substances absorbed from the mother's bloodstream. These substances that interfere with the development of the fetus are called teratogens. The most critical period comes early in the pregnancy, in the first 18 to 60 days. This is an especially troublesome problem because some women are unaware they are pregnant during this time. Furthermore, damaging teratogens can cross over the placenta—the membrane organ that connects the embryo to the food and oxygen supply of the mother—in amounts that apparently may not affect the mother's health or sense of well-being at that stage.

One of the most widely publicized teratogens in recent years is Thalidomide. This drug, administered to women to combat nausea, caused widespread birth defects. Most heavy metals, such as lead, mercury or

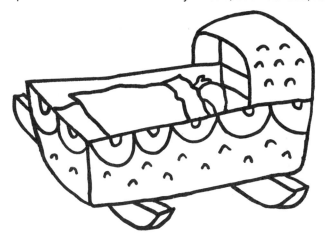

cadmium, can have teratogenic effects. In other publicized cases, some companies which use lead in their operations have barred women from working in lead-related jobs.

In addition to birth defects, toxic substances that affect the germ cells (mutagens) or the fetus (teratogens) can result in miscarriages or still-births.

Work-related miscarriages, or spontaneous abortion, usually occur fairly early in the pregnancy. During the first 18 to 60 days, the major organ systems are being developed in the fetus. The damage done at this stage may be so extensive that the fetus cannot survive, resulting usually in miscarriage. An increased number of spontaneous abortions has been noted in women who work around anesthetics in operating rooms and dental clinics.

After birth, workplace hazards can continue to pose health problems for children. The Coalition for the Reproductive Rights of Workers (CRROW) reports the case of a 6-week-old baby poisoned by breast milk contaminated by a dry-cleaning solvent which the mother inhaled during regular lunchtime visits with her husband at the plant. The infant developed a liver disease, but improved after the mother stopped breast feeding.

CRROW also notes that higher levels of birth defects have been recorded in communities located near petrochemical plants and places where vinyl chloride is used. Asbestos dust and pesticides may be brought into the home from work, raising another risk for young children.

Much more information about this vital subject is needed. More testing needs to be done on chemicals and physical agents that can interfere with the right to bear and raise healthy children. In the meantime, in the words of the Coalition for the Reproductive Rights of Workers: "No one knows the workplace better than the worker. In the case of reproductive hazards, as in any other health and safety problem, it is up to the worker to discover the hazard and work for its elimination."

Job Poisons & the Male Sex Role

One of the less talked about and, until fairly recently, less studied occupational hazards for male workers relates to the reproductive system. Most of our concerns in the past were directed toward women in the workforce who may have had trouble conceiving, or experiencing normal pregnancy and childbirth—problems brought on or made worse by their occupational environment. Now, researchers are beginning to pay closer attention to how the male sex drive and reproductive function can be interfered with by exposure to certain toxins.

The testes and sperm are particularly susceptible to damage. There was a forewarning of this possibility in situations outside the workplace. Physicians treating cancer patients with chemotherapy have long been aware of testicular dysfunction associated with this form of treatment. However, only recently has testicular dysfunction been studied in connection with occupational exposure to chemical toxins.

One of these toxins is the pesticide DBCP, used to control nematodes. Overexposure to the chemical has been associated with irreversible azospermia, a condition in which the semen contains no sperm. This means that a man so afflicted cannot become a natural father.

Azospermia, incidentally, is not the same as impotence—the inability to have sexual intercourse. However, the condition might have some psychological effect on the man which might hinder, perhaps temporarily, his sexual activity. DBCP is known to be carcinogenic—capable of producing cancer—in laboratory animals. But it is not clear at this time to what extent genetic damage is involved in DBCP toxicity. So, exactly how the chemical works to injure the male reproductive system must be considered unknown.

Reduced sperm counts have been reported among workers severely poisoned by kepone.

Carbon disulfide is a question mark. One study of workers exposed to carbon disulfide showed reductions in sperm counts, and alterations in the structure of the sperm. Yet a larger study, conducted by the National Institute for Occupational Safety and Health (NIOSH), did not reveal any seminal abnormalities.

Many metals widely used in industry are believed to be reproductive system poisons. Mercury, not surprisingly, is prominent on the list. Mercury compounds have been used for many years as intravaginal contraceptives.

A study in Romania reported infertility and loss of libido (sex drive) in lead workers. Many of these workers also showed some nerve damage. This study has not been confirmed in the United States, but the Romanian findings are consistent with experimental evidence of hormonal derangement caused by lead exposure.

Cadmium, nickel and methyl mercury have been shown to cause damage to the testicles of laboratory animals. Zinc, cadmium and mercury alter the proteins in the sperm of sea urchins.

Animal experiments also have turned up reproductive abnormalities caused by certain non-metals. These include organotin, DDT, DDVP, ethylene dibromide, and metanil yellow. Spontaneous abortions in wives of men exposed on the job to anaesthetic gases and vinyl chloride point to these substances as possible sources of genetic damage in the husbands.

133

Men also should be aware that industrial chemicals and metals are not the only suspected culprits. Some of the most common and widely used recreational substances may have undesirable effects on reproduction. Excessive alcohol consumption is a well-known cause of impotence. It may heighten the urge, but it can lower the performance. Decreased levels of testosterone (the male sex hormone) and low sperm counts have been reported in marijuana smokers.

And stress, certainly, has an adverse effect on one's sex life.

As you may have noticed, a number of the experiments mentioned here are based on animal studies in laboratories. While highly useful, this information needs to be correlated with data from vitally needed human studies which, so far, are lacking or are sketchy at best. We need much more awareness in this field—for the sake of healthy, happy family relationships, and for future generations.

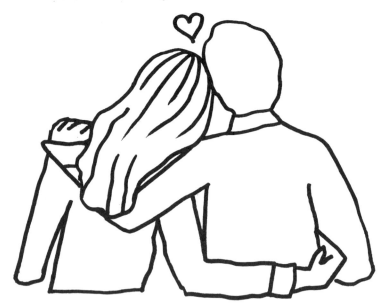

On-the-Job 'Heart Poisons'

The Big Three risk factors in heart disease, most experts agree, are:
- Cigarette smoking;
- Elevated levels of cholesterol in the blood; and
- Hypertension (high blood pressure).

But are there other risk factors—cardiotoxins, or "heart poisons"—in the workplace and the environment that can aggravate or trigger the deadly effects of the Big Three? So far, that question hasn't received the attention it deserves from researchers. It's time it did. These other risk factors may include chemicals and heavy metals, gases, fibrogenic dusts and physical agents. Some evidence already suggests that hydrocarbons and fluorocarbons can cause changes in the heart's rhythm. Heart tissue damage has been noticed in cases involving exposure to cobalt, antimony, arsenic and yellow phosphorus. Patients being treated with antimony for parasites have shown changes in their electrocardiograms, according to some investigators.

Cadmium levels in the air seem to have some connection with cardiovascular death rates. We know that cadmium is present in cigarette smoke, and that smokers have increased levels of cadmium in their blood. But the connection is still not clear and needs more study.

Other clues suggest that lead is responsible for raising cholesterol levels in the blood. Typesetters and compositors exposed to lead and antimony fumes show an increased cardiovascular death rate compared with other printing crafts. Other workers exposed to lead include painters and paint makers, welders and battery workers.

Carbon disulfide, a gas widely used in the manufacture of rubber and synthetic fibers, can result in hypertension. It is also suspected of raising the level of cholesterol in the blood. Studies show that workers exposed to carbon disulfide have twice the risk of heart disease as those not exposed to the gas. People who work with carbon disulfide include degreasers, dry cleaners, electroplaters, rayon makers and rubber workers.

Carbon monoxide is another gas that has shown the potential for increasing cholesterol deposits and aggravating other vascular conditions. Government studies suggest that carbon monoxide may add to hardening of the arteries (artherosclerosis). It can do this because it is able to penetrate the tissue that lines blood vessels, the lymphatic system, and various fluid-bathed cavities of the body.

The connection between inhaled fibrogenic dusts and lung diseases is well established. But any relationship between lung diseases and the subsequent development of heart disease is not yet so clear-cut. However, we do know that with sufficient exposure, a certain percentage of lung-damaged individuals will be so severely affected that right-sided heart failure is likely to occur.

Noise, heat and cold are physical agents. All are associated with job stress. Deadlines, quotas, responsibility for others—these are also job stress factors, although, strictly speaking, not "physical agents."

The experts are still debating the question of whether stress can make you sick. But a number of studies have shown that people in high-stress jobs have higher blood pressures, higher cholesterol levels, and more heart attacks than those in low-stress occupations.

Nerve Poisons

Talk about nerve poisons in the workplace and some people think of science fiction, or horror movies, or the dark secrets of chemical warfare. But neurotoxins are not new and exotic. And they are a lot more common than many workers realize.

Before Christ, lead and smelter laborers complained of tingling and numbness in their hands and feet. They became confused. Some went blind.

Less than 100 years ago in England, iron bars were sometimes placed over the windows of vulcanizing rooms in rubber factories. They weren't there to keep out burglars. They were there to keep workers from jumping out during fits of madness.

And only about 10 years ago, workers in a Columbus, Ohio, fabric-coating plant began to experience a puzzling weakness of the hands and feet. They found it hard to do such simple things as turning a key, using a screwdriver, flipping a switch. Some walked with a peculiar slapping gait. Others had trouble walking at all.

These were all victims of neurotoxins at work over the centuries. Today, an estimated 20 million Americans work with one or more chemicals known to be neurotoxic. The National Institute for Occupational Safety and Health (NIOSH) lists 163 chemicals (out of some 100,000 or more used by industry) as dangerous enough to carry a recommended Threshold Limit Value (TLV) of exposure. An additional 43 chemicals have TLVs because they can cause secondary nerve and behavioral effects.

Most of these chemicals are organic solvents, either from coal tar or petroleum, and include such substances as benzene, toluene, xylene, chlorinated hydrocarbons, alcohols, acetones and ketones among others. The Ohio outbreak was caused by ketone which, up to that time, was thought to be a fairly harmless ink thinner and machinery cleaner.

Organic solvents are used to make paints, varnishes, plastics, synthetic textiles, rubber, explosives and dyes. They also show up in such consumer products as aerosol sprays, shoe polish, household cleaners and seat cushions.

Certain metals, such as lead, mercury and manganese, can also cause nerve damage. Carbon monoxide is another large potential source of neurotoxicity because of the widespread use of combustion processes in industry.

Cardiotoxins—heart poisons—need more study because heart attacks, strokes, high blood pressure and other forms of cardiovascular disease account for half of all deaths in this country. In economic terms, more than 50 million man-days a year are lost because of these diseases of the heart and blood vessels. The cost to workers is a staggering 30 percent of all health care costs.

The Body's Skin Surface

"Skin?" The bright kid pondered the question. "It's what holds the rest of me inside."

That's how a lot of people think of this remarkable covering of the body—as a sort of flexible envelope for the skeleton, muscles, fat, organs, nerves, fluids and so on that make up a human being. Actually, the skin is an organ—the largest organ of the body. It makes up the largest surface area in close contact with foreign substances in nature as well as in the industrial environment. And, not surprising in light of this, occupational skin disease is our most common industrial illness.

Since organic solvents are hungry for fats, the nervous system and its sheath-like defenses are particularly vulnerable to attack. The poisons enter the body chiefly by inhalation. Toxic effects generally result from chronic exposure and may go undetected for long periods of time.

Typically, nerve poisoning gives its first warning as a tingling and numbness of the hands and feet. Over time—often as long as years—other symptoms may develop if the exposure continues. These symptoms might take a variety of forms: tremors, lack of coordination, paralysis, impotence, sensory damage, lowered alertness, loss of memory, irritability, depression, hallucination and so on.

Prolonged hospitalization or therapy may be required in some cases. Irreversible damage occurs in a significant number of victims. Since the central nervous system cannot replace lost cells, damage to the central memory and intellectual control functions is essentially permanent.

Regulating neurotoxins is largely covered by three laws: the Toxic Substances Control Act (TOSCA) and the Clean Air Act, both administered by the Environmental Protection Agency (EPA), and the Occupational Safety and Health Act, administered by OSHA.

But laws—no matter how well intentioned—are only as effective as the willingness to enforce them. And this commitment to workers' safety today falls far short of what is needed, and what was intended by those who wrote the laws.

Workers and their unions need to be alert to every hazard, and to insist on strict compliance with every safeguard, adding new ones as the needs arise. Anything less is not enough to prevent a pattern of personal tragedy that is centuries old.

At any given time, one in a hundred workers will show some form of occupational dermatosis. That means more than 1 million people in a workforce of over 100 million are suffering from a discoloration, a blemish, a callous, an inflammatory eruption or a tumor.

A California study a few years ago showed that at least one-third of all compensated industrial diseases involved a skin problem. And that doesn't include thousands of cases of dermatitis—that's the inflammatory form of dermatosis—which are not compensated because workers don't lose time from work.

Healthy skin serves you in five main ways:

1. It protects.
2. It helps to regulate body temperature.
3. It senses—helps you feel things.
4. It absorbs.
5. It manufactures some of its own protective substances.

Certain layers block the entrance of water and water-soluble chemicals. Color and thickness guard against the effects of sunlight and other sources of physical energy. The whole elastic shield protects underlying muscles, nerves and blood vessels.

Working with the blood vessels and nerves, the skin helps to regulate body temperature. It does this by sweating. As the sweat evaporates, surface heat is dissipated, keeping the blood in the enlarged vessels at a relatively constant temperature. Conversely, if the body is exposed to severe cold, the skin's blood vessels contract to conserve heat.

The skin is laced with nerve endings and fibers. This network makes up a sensing system that lets you tell the difference between hot and cold, wet and dry, thick and thin, rough and smooth, hard and soft.

The skin's ability to absorb is a source of both benefit and hazard. On the one hand, it allows dry skin to replenish lost moisture. On the other hand, absorption opens the way for potentially harmful substances to break through the defense mechanisms. Cuts, hair follicles and the spaces around skin hairs are the most likely entry points. The skin also permits ready exchange of gases, except for carbon monoxide.

The major manufactured products of the skin are pigment and an oily substance called sebum. Pigment gives the skin its color and acts as a partial sunscreen. Exactly how the body uses sebum is unclear. But when it is present in normal amounts, it helps to provide some surface protection.

Sebum forms a waxy emulsion that slows down the entrance of water and water-soluble chemicals. This emulsion layer is easily removed by soap, solvents and alkalis, but comes back naturally.

Below this protective emulsion is the keratin layer consisting of dead cells that are constantly produced and shed as part of the normal life of

138

the skin. Sebum helps to break down keratin and sweat, probably help-ing the body's renewal processes. Keratin moderately resists mild acids and water, but is susceptible to the actions of alkali, strong detergents, solvents and prolonged exposure to warm water. Ultraviolet light causes the layer to thicken.

The lower portion of the keratin layer contains an important barrier that prevents marked loss of water and the wholesale entrance of water-soluble materials. It can be altered by injury, strong chemical agents, solvents or internal diseases which disrupt the skin.

This thin, incredibly complex outer surface we present to the world is far more than just a body-sized glove. It is a flexible envelope that keeps all our other parts inside, as the youngster said. It is a vital, but vulnerable organ—the largest we have.

Occupational Skin Diseases

Skin diseases are the most frequently reported occupational illnesses.

- Two out of every 1,000 California workers a year reported a skin dis-ease in a recent compilation of the state's department of industrial relations. That's 17,000 cases in industries covered by the California Workers' Compensation Act (8.5 million persons).
- Women accounted for 28 percent of all reported cases, although they make up more than 40 percent of California's workforce.
- In manufacturing, however, women had a higher incidence rate of skin disease than men, 4.7 per 1,000, compared to 3.8 for men.
- Agricultural workers were four times as likely to get a job-related skin disease as workers in general, 8.6 per 1,000 compared to 2.1.
- Physicians expect 1 out of 5 workers with an occupational skin condi-tion to lose some time from work. The average time lost is about nine workdays.
- One out of 10 workers with a disabling dermatitis had been on the job one month or less.
- Most occupational skin diseases show up in the summer or early fall.

Generally, occupational skin problems can be traced to one or more of three main causes: chemical agents, physical factors and biological agents.

Chemical agents. These cause most problems, either by irritating the skin or sensitizing it. Primary irritants damage normal skin on contact, depending on how strong the concentration is and how long the contact lasts. These substances include inorganic acids, alkalis, heavy metal salts, tanning agents, bleaches and chlorine compounds. About 80 percent of all occupational skin diseases are caused by primary irritants. The other 20 percent are due to sensitized or allergic reactions. Almost any chemical and certain plants—poison ivy or oak, for example—can cause this type of allergic dermatitis. But a person must have been exposed to the active agent—sensitized—at least once previously before the dermatitis will appear. The time period can range from five to seven days or more. Occasionally, months or years may go by before a worker who is continually exposed to a specific agent will develop an allergic eruption.

Sensitizers are found in certain dyes, rubber ingredients, unfinished plastics, and such metals as nickel, chrome and mercury.

Physical factors. These include excessive heat, cold, sunlight, ionizing radiation and artifical ultraviolet light. Artificial ultraviolet light is produced by hot metals, welding and the plasma torch. It can cause burns. Excessive exposure to X rays and radioactive materials can produce severe damage to the skin, or to the entire body.

Biological agents. A generalized disease process can come about through bacterial, fungal and parasitic infections of the skin. Animal handlers, packinghouse workers, hide handlers, kitchen employees, agricultural workers, bakers, florists, nursery workers and laboratory technicians are among those who may be affected by such agents. Likewise, wood workers, lumberjacks, electric lineworkers and road builders are exposed to a number of plants and timber which irritate the skin.

Other factors—usually beyond an individual's control—seem to give certain people a built-in tendency to break out with something when others are not affected. These factors include the sex of the person, age, skin color (light or dark), texture (thick, thin), type (oily, dry), or a history of allergy.

Another factor that can adversely affect a person's susceptibility to skin disease (and one certainly within each individual's control) is personal cleanliness.

Occupational dermatitis is a preventable disease. The best way to keep it in check is through engineering controls at the worksite. Ideally, the factory layout and equipment should protect workers from contact with potentially hazardous substances. If the hazard can't be closed off entirely, other controls should collect and take out irritating dusts, vapors, fumes and mists.

Washing hands, wearing clean work clothes and keeping clean on the job is every worker's responsibility. Adequate washing facilities must be available and supplied with good cleansing materials. Washing should be done before and after lunch, before breaks and at the end of the shift. Some jobs may be so unclean that more frequent washing, even showers, may be required.

Protective clothing should be provided by the employer. That's one way to make sure it's worn and kept in good condition. Also, it prevents a worker's family from being contaminated since the work clothes don't have to be taken home to be washed.

Not only is the skin the body's largest organ; it makes up the largest area exposed to foreign substances in nature as well as the industrial environment. Taking care of it properly is, literally, a first line of defense for your general health.

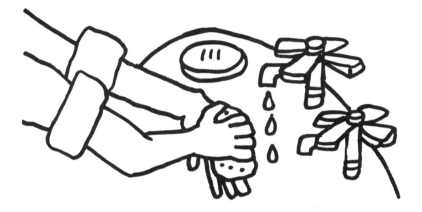

How to Handle Burn Injuries

Despite continuing programs of education and prevention, more than 2 million persons suffer burn injuries each year. Of that number, about 12,000 die and some 50,000 require hospitalization from six weeks to two years. These figures and some of the following material are based on an article by Madeleine T. Martin, MSN, Project Director, Burn and Trauma Nursing, University of Cincinnati, which appeared in *Occupational Safety and Health.*

Unlike other types of injury accidents that happen and then stop—such as falls or the impact of heavy objects—burns keep on going until stopped by the victim or somebody nearby. So the first rule in responding to a burn accident is speed—with caution.

Separate the victim from the heat source as quickly as possible. Smother the flames. Break the electrical current. Wash the chemical or scald with large amounts of cool water. These are the major types of industrial burns. In the case of fire, smoldering clothing should be removed along with any metallic objects that retain heat, such as rings or belt buckles. However, clothing that sticks to the skin should only be dampened to cool the heat and left in place for removal at the hospital.

In the case of electrical injuries, there is another immediate emergency action that may be called for: Make sure breathing is maintained. The cardiopulmonary system—the heart and lungs—is especially vulnerable to cardiac and respiratory arrest, demanding immediate resuscitation.

A prompt assessment of the injury should determine the percentage of body surface affected, the depth of tissue damage, and the type of agent that caused the burn—flame, electricity, chemical or whatever. This will help to indicate the proper on-the-spot first aid treatment or, if the injury is more extensive, how to prepare the victim for transfer to a hospital or burn center.

Generally, the larger the burned area, the more serious the injury. The depth of tissue destruction is designated either partial or full thickness. Partial thickness refers to the skin and the thin layer of cells underneath—provided enough of the underlying cells remain undamaged to provide for spontaneous healing. However, these partial thickness burns can become full thickness if infection causes further destruction. Partial burns characteristically appear red.

Full thickness burns involve not only destruction of the skin and thin layer underneath, but go down to the underlying fat, and may include muscle and bone tissue. Appearance can range from cherry red to gray or black; the surface can vary from wet to dry and leathery. Healing does not take place spontaneously and grafting may be required to cover the wound.

Electrical burns can be deceptive because skin damage may be seen only at the point of contact, entry or exit. But deep and extensive damage may occur because the body acts as a conductor from the source of the electricity to the ground, generating deep thermal destruction.

Chemical burns are caused by substances that are either primarily acid or alkaline. Acids cause damage by interacting with and coagulating tissue, that is by changing a liquid or soft solid into a semi-hard or hard mass, like blood clotting or a scab forming. In some cases, this may act to seal off the wound and prevent deeper damage. Alkalines, on the other hand, have somewhat opposite actions. They tend to liquify tissue and allow for deeper penetration.

Immediate treatment for chemical accidents, in most cases, involves flushing the affected areas with large amounts of water to remove the substance. However, this may not be the case with some chemicals. The plant nurse or designated first aid person should know the specific chemicals used in the workplace and the recommended first aid treatment for these special agents.

Minor burns, in which the area is less than 10 percent partial thickness or 2 percent full thickness, can usually be treated at the workplace, in a physician's office, or in an emergency room on an out-patient basis. These would not include burns involving the eyes, face, hands, feet or crotch areas. These should be treated as more serious injuries, regardless of the extent of the burns.

Moderate burns of 10 to 20 percent partial and less than 10 percent full thickness generally require hospitalization. Severe burns, where more than 20 percent of the body is affected by partial and more than 10 percent by full thickness injuries, should be treated at a special burn care center.

In all cases, if electricity, inhalation or multiple injuries are involved, the victim should be treated in a facility staffed and equipped to handle severe burns.

Low Back Pain

Backache, or low back pain, just misses falling into the category of human afflictions that some people find funny—like gout—until it hits them. Then they find out quickly and sharply that back pain is not a laughing matter. In the first place, there's just too much of it "going around."

Of the 25 million to 35 million persons classified as chronically disabled by the National Institute of Handicapped Research, about 8 million suffer from chronic low back pain; about 1 million are unable to work. Among Americans under age 45, back impairment is the single most common disability, and it ranks third among the 45 and 65 age group, just behind heart disease and arthritis. In 1978, low back injuries accounted for 25 million lost work-days and $14 billion was spent in the treatment of industrial back injuries.

So back pain is more than just an individual misery for millions. It is a crippling national problem as well.

The causes of the many different kinds of low back pain are too numerous to go into here. They can range from tumors to infections; from metabolic disease to pelvic disorders. And that doesn't begin to cover the whole list. Here I am going to talk mostly about causes that working men and women are familiar with: chronic or acute strains or sprains. And we can narrow this even further by talking about just two activities—lifting and sitting.

To get a better picture of what we are talking about, think of your back as a stack of somewhat circular building blocks. Between each of these blocks, which are bone, are discs made up of a firm outer ring and a soft center. These discs help hold the backbones together and act as shock absorbers.

When you bend or twist this flexible column, the backbones exert pressure on the outer edges of the cushioning rings or discs. Swedish scientists have found that simply bending from the waist with the legs straight can generate more than 200 pounds per square inch inside the back.

Trouble begins when small cracks develop in the outer ring of the discs. We find this condition reaches a peak between the ages of 35 and 55. If the pressure is too great, the outer ring can bulge or even rupture. And this can let the soft center ooze out like toothpaste from a tube. When this soft material touches a nerve, you feel a sharp pain or spasm.

With this picture in mind, let's consider a step-by-step way to lift safely and minimize these possibly injurious pressures:

1. Place your feet close to the object to be lifted so you don't have to lean forward. The feet should be 8 to 12 inches apart for good balance.
2. Bend the knees to the degree that is comfortable for you to get a good handhold. Then using both back and leg muscles, lift the load straight up, smoothly and evenly. Push with your legs and keep the load close to your body.
3. Don't make any turning or twisting movements until you have lifted the load into a carrying position. Then, when you want to make a move in the direction you want to go, do so by changing the direction of your feet; not by twisting your body first.

Setting the load down is just as important as picking it up. Using your leg and back muscles, comfortably lower the load by bending your knees. When the load is securely in position release your grip, then straighten your knees until you are upright again.

Back problems caused by sitting are usually caused by a poorly designed chair, stool or workbench. There are three key factors to look for in a well-designed chair: height; backrest; seat.

The right height for you when seated is for the hips and knees to be at right angles when your feet are flat on the floor. The backrest should fit snugly into the small of your back to support the spine and lower back. You should be able to adjust it forward or backward so the size of the seat is right for you.

The seat should slant backward just enough to allow you to lean comfortably against the backrest, but not slip so deeply into the chair that you have to stretch and strain to reach things. A well-fitting seat will end about five inches from the crease behind your knees when you are sitting aginst the backrest. Textured fabric seat coverings are better than vinyl or other plastics because they keep you from sliding forward.

Low back pain, from whatever causes, is disabling and costly both in terms of absenteeism as well as decreased productivity on the job. Edu-

144

cational programs have proved helpful in reducing this problem. Good liaison between the occupational physician and the employee's personal physician can do much to ease anxieties and fears and contribute to overall better labor relations.

'Sprain' or 'Strain'—Take Care

"Say Joe, when you pull a muscle, do you say 'strain' or 'sprain'? " asked Alice, who was nursing a sore wrist.

"Neither," Joe grinned. "I say 'ouch!' "

Joking aside, what is the difference between a strain and a sprain? A strain, generally, is an injury caused by excessive stretching or overuse of a muscle or connecting tissue (tendons) where no joint is involved. A sprain is an injury caused by severe stretching of the tough bands of tissue (ligaments), usually around joints.

Tendons are like cords that connect a muscle to bone. Ligaments are like bands that connect bone to bone, or hold organs in place. Ligaments keep our joints together while permitting movement. So, you "sprain" your wrist (ankle, elbow, shoulder, etc). But you "strain" your eyes if you misuse them. Sprains, as a rule, are more serious than strains.

Treatment of most mild to moderate strains and sprains consists of elevating the affected part, resting it, and applying ice or cold compresses to help reduce swelling. An elastic bandage is good for support.

You can get a strain or sprain in countless ways—from careless lifting to tripping over a curb; from an automobile accident to an athletic mishap. However it happens, you'll feel pain. There'll be tenderness at the point of injury. There'll probably be swelling. And, in more severe cases, discoloration. Both types of injury can put you out of commission for awhile. How long will depend on how severely you have overtaxed the tendon or ligament involved.

In sprains, particularly, the ligament may be partially or completely torn. The joint may become unstable. In that case, it may be necessary to immobilize the limb in a compression bandage or cast. Where a ligament has been partially torn—say at the ankle or knee—you should put only minimal weight on the affected limb for three days. Crutches help. If the ligament is completely torn, you shouldn't put any weight on the injured part for three days at least. If immobilizing the limb doesn't work, surgery may be required to mend the tear in severe cases.

Because they are such common injuries, both on and off the job, strains and sprains may be taken too lightly. This isn't a good idea for an important reason a lot of people don't appreciate. It is not always

145

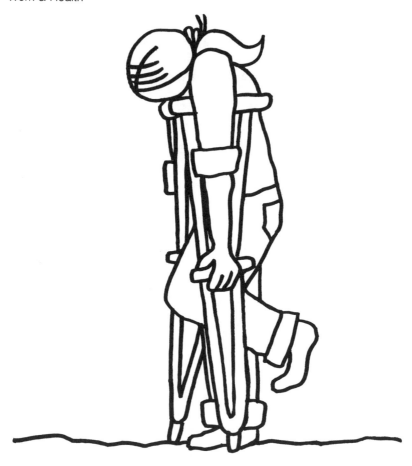

easy to tell whether you've simply overstretched a muscle, tendon or ligament, or whether you've broken a bone. Both fractures and sprains have several similar symptoms: pain, swelling, and limited motion.

If you're not sure what has happened, play it safe and treat the injury as a fracture until a medical examination proves otherwise. Fractures range all the way from a hairline crack to a complete break. If the injury is so severe that the broken end of the bone punctures the skin, it is called a compound fracture. That's the one case you won't confuse with a sprain.

In a bone break, as in some severe sprains, there may be deformity, such as an arm or leg that appears to have been forced into an unnatural position, and can't be straightened. There may be loss of mobility, loss of power, or even a grating noise between the fractured ends.

Obviously, an injury severe enough to break a bone will damage other tissue. The first order of business is to limit the damage. That means limiting further movement. If no trained medical help is available, you can immobilize a broken limb by making a splint from a board or roll of newspaper. Tie it in place, but not too tightly. If there is bleeding, apply a pressure bandage directly to the site. If you suspect that the spine or neck is involved, don't move the victim at all. Get professional medical help immediately.

"Do not further damage" is one of the first things medical students are taught. It's a good lesson to remember if you're unlucky enough to feel that sudden jolt of lightning pain in a muscle or joint—whether you say "strain" or "sprain" or "ouch!" By whatever name, all injuries need to be treated, above all, with respect.

Allergies

The word allergy means "altered reaction." If you're allergic to something, it means that your body reacts differently—and uncomfortably—to a substance that doesn't bother other people.

Substances that cause allergic reactions are known as allergens or antigens. They can be grouped into four categories, depending on whether you breathe them, swallow them, touch them or are injected with them:

- *Inhalant allergens* include pollens from grasses, plants and trees; dust, mold spores, fungi, dog and cat dander, tobacco, etc.
- *Ingestants,* those that get in by mouth, include eggs, chicken, chocolate, nuts, shellfish, pork, milk, strawberries, aspirin and antibiotics.
- *Contactants* are such touchables as dyes, poison ivy, nylon, certain metals (like nickel), cosmetics and wool.
- *Injectants* enter through a skin puncture, such as a penicillin shot or bee or wasp sting.

These are just a few of what may be countless allergens or antigens.

Normally, when harmful germs enter the body, various defense mechanisms spring into action and produce antibodies to destroy or neutralize the foreign invaders.

In an allergic situation, however, the body's defense response is abnormal. It reacts to the foreign invaders by producing allergic antibodies to meet a threat that the non-allergic person's body may simply shrug off. These allergic antibodies dash into the fray to do battle with the invading allergens. In the melee, certain chemicals are released by the body's cells. Among these chemical compounds are histamine and bradykinin.

Histamine can cause swelling of the mucous membranes of the nose and itching of the eyes, producing watery discharges. Do those symptoms sound familiar? That's right—hay fever.

Bradykinin can cause smooth muscles like those in the walls of the small tubes in the lungs to squeeze down, trapping air. The effort of trying to expel the air produces the wheezing noise associated with asthma.

As you might expect, the inhaled allergens produce symptoms in the nose and lungs. Those that enter by the mouth can produce headaches, rashes and gastrointestinal symptoms. Allergens in the "touch" category generally show up as skin problems—nettle rashes, eczema, dermatitis and so on. To confuse the situation even further, the same allergens may cause different reactions in different people.

Allergic reactions like hay fever and asthma tend to run in families. One study has shown that 80 percent of hay fever sufferers have a family history of the allergy. If both parents are allergic, more than half of their children are likely to be allergic.

However, it sometimes happens that the tendency to an allergy may skip a generation and then recur. And, although the tendency is inherited, the specific allergy may not be. A parent may have hay fever and the child asthma.

Many people with contact dermatitis have no personal or family history of any allergies. One day, the skin reaction just appears. Actually, it may have taken a year or two of exposure to a specific substance for the allergic response to develop. The first step in treatment is to identify and remove the responsible allergens. Sometimes, that's not so easy—especially in certain jobs. In such cases, barrier creams, gloves and protective clothing are called for.

About one person in six is severely allergic to the venom from the stings of bees and wasps. Where most people experience only a localized and somewhat painful swelling after a sting, the hypersensitive person may react with generalized hives, fainting, abdominal pains and breathing difficulties. If you have had such severe symptoms, see your doctor.

Few allergies are ever "cured." In most cases, avoiding the allergens that cause the difficulties holds the best promise for the allergic person to make life more comfortable.

Hay fever sufferers and asthmatics often find relief by sleeping and working in an air conditioned environment where temperature and humidity are under control and pollens and molds are kept out. Dust should be reduced to a minimum.

With some allergies, it may be necessary to get rid of a family pet, or cut out certain foods and medication. You may have to avoid certain materials in clothing, or change your brand of cosmetics. Drastic reactions may require a job change.

Medically supervised injections of specific allergens to desensitize patients is a lengthy process and sometimes produces disappointing results. Research is going forward in this area and progress is being made. Various medications often provide temporary relief. One of the most widely used is antihistamines. But, here again, the results are spotty, and what may help one sufferer may do little or nothing for another.

Allergic management boils down to medical detective work. You can help by working with your doctor to pinpoint your own specific "who-done-it."

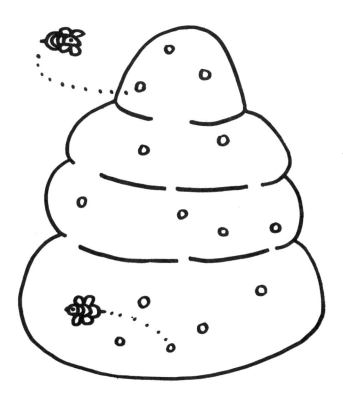

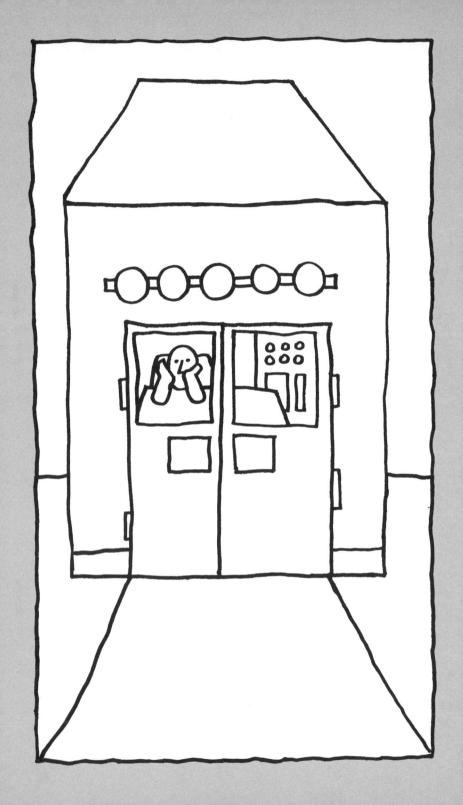

6 Controlling Job Hazards

Job Health through Engineering

The most effective and permanent way to control health hazards in the workplace is by using engineering controls. There are three principal types of such controls: substitution, isolation and ventilation. Here are some examples of each of these techniques.

Substitution. Substitution is the most positive of all engineering controls. If a material, machine or process is dangerous, the best control is one that replaces any one or all of those hazardous factors.

An example of a material substitution is the case of vinyl chloride, which was being used in paint aerosol cans until it was found to cause liver cancer. Carbon dioxide was found to be a good replacement as a propellent.

Diesel forktrucks, which produce high levels of carbon monoxide (CO) can be replaced with propane-driven trucks which run much cleaner and give off less CO. That's an example of mechanical substitution.

Process substitution made the work environment safer in a plant that was spray painting metal sheets after fabrication. This caused inhalation hazards because of the mist and vapor. This hazard was substantially reduced by pre-coating the sheets at a permanent, well-ventilated dip tank.

Isolation. Isolation of a hazard means putting some kind of barrier between you and the hazard. Distance is an effective barrier in some cases. Noise is a good example of a potential hazard that can be dealt with in a number of ways through engineering controls.

Physically, noise consists of pressure vibrations in a medium—the air for example. In other words, sound is a form of energy, and this energy can be dampened by:

- Putting sound-absorbing material around a noisy machine.
- Isolating a machine by putting it on resilient vibration mountings to absorb the energy before it is transformed into noise.
- Isolating workers in soundproof booths.
- Setting up the work station at a safe distance from the noisy machinery. A safe distance is where the noise level is less than 80

decibels. This distance can be located by determining the noise levels at various distances from the source of the noise by using a sound level meter.

Ventilation. Ventilation means moving the air to keep contaminants— dusts, mists, gases, fumes or vapors—from reaching the breathing zone of workers. There are two kinds of ventilation: general or dilution, and local exhaust.

General or dilution ventilation provides a constant exchange of air in a room. Thus, it dilutes contaminants that may be in that room. This type of ventilation works well in offices and other work areas where the air needs to be exchanged to make it fresher. However, it offers little protection when the air contains toxic materials.

Local exhaust ventilation is the only way to control air contamination at the source. When engineered properly, it will capture the contaminants before they can escape and enter the worker's breathing zone.

In the case of some chemicals covered by federal health standards, engineering controls are required by law to protect workers. If the exposure is more than that allowed by a particular standard or limit, the employer must develop a plan to reduce the exposure by using engineering controls.

Workers are entitled to see these plans. You can exercise your rights by letting the Occupational Safety and Health Administration's industrial hygienists know that you and your designated representative wish to be informed of any employer abatement plans that are submitted to OSHA. You and your representative can petition the court for the third-party status in abatement plan proceedings.

Controlling Toxic Fumes

Harriet M. is a 36-year-old woman who works as a meat wrapper in a chain supermarket. She likes her job. The pay is good; the hours and working conditions are agreeable. She gets along with her fellow workers. But Harriet lately has been complaining of a persistent cough, chest tightness and shortness of breath. She thought it might be from the frequent exposure to cold air when the butchers opened the doors of the meat storage and cutting room.

Actually, Harriet is suffering from an occupationally related condition— a form of asthma associated with meat wrapping.

Let's look closely at her job. The thin, clear plastic wrapping Harriet uses to cover the meats before they are put in the cases out front for sale is a material called polyvinyl chloride (PVC). Harriet works at a machine which cuts the material to size with a hot wire and seals it with a heated flat plate. The temperatures are around 140 to 160 degrees Fahrenheit. This heat causes the plastic to release fumes or vapors into the air. Fumes are also produced in the adhesive labeling process.

In general, we believe that the heat removes some of the water content of the polyvinyl chloride to produce gaseous chemical products such as hydrogen chloride, benzylchloride, possibly phosgene and other complex byproducts. Phosgene also may be found where increased carbon monoxide is present due to inadequate ventilation.

In all of these situations, the fumes generated by the effect of heat on the plastic are worsened and complicated by cigarette smoking.

Recent studies have shown that 67 percent of the workers exposed to the heating process in meat wrapping and labeling complain of one or more of these symptoms: coughing, chest tightness, wheezing, shortness of breath and chest pain.

When workers show symptoms like these—and there is no family history of asthma—there is a strong suspicion that something in the occupational setting is to blame. The breathing difficulties can develop in some sensitive persons almost immediately. In others, the troublesome symptoms may not show up until several hours after exposure.

Now, perhaps you think the case of Harriet M. is too specialized for you to worry about. After all, meat wrapping is a very small job classification in the whole range of occupations. But let's enlarge the picture. Suppose you work in a situation where you can inhale a toxic substance, whether it comes from plastic wrapping or anything else. What can you do to reduce such hazards?

A first step is to get the work area monitored. This should be done frequently by the employer on a continuing basis in order to set up proper preventive measures. The primary goal is early detection of occupational toxicants for the total prevention of adverse health effects. The long-range goal is to keep the working environment safe once the trouble has been located and taken care of.

Not all workers exposed to toxic inhalants will be affected the same way or in the same length of time. The effects are modified by a number of factors—the body's natural resistance in different individuals, the size of the inhaled particles, how long these agents stay in the breathing apparatus and so on.

In addition to frequent industrial hygiene monitoring and early detection of the offending material, there are other steps that can be taken to manage the situation. These include:

- Use of appropriate dust and respiratory masks.
- Adequate ventilation of the worksite.

- Complete cessation of tobacco smoke exposure.
- Vaccination (influenza and pneumonia-type vaccines are sometimes used).
- Getting away from the harmful exposure as quickly as possible; this is particularly important for hypersensitive people who are severely affected.

Plastic wrapping of meat and other food products undoubtedly has been a boon for the consumer. But it has come at a potential price for some sensitive workers in the form of occupational asthma. Fortunately, the risk can be minimized by good industrial hygienic practices at the worksite, and by the use of personal protective devices.

Personal Protective Equipment

Personal protective equipment can help to keep you from being hurt on the job, or getting sick from conditions you work under, or from the materials you handle. Important? Yes. The best way? No.

The best on-the-job protection starts with the plant itself, with safe machinery, clean air, efficient layout and work flow, proper handling procedures for dangerous materials, control over the time you may be exposed to a hazardous situation, and reduced noise.

It's within that total picture that personal protective equipment must be considered.

The big drawback to personal protective equipment is that it doesn't reduce or eliminate the hazard. If your equipment fails, you are immediately unprotected. Nevertheless, it is important to understand how and when and why you may need to protect yourself. Here are some points to keep in mind about personal protective equipment:

1. It's got to work. There's nothing more useless than a piece of equipment that's supposed to protect you and doesn't do the job. Strange as it may seem, too often workers are given equipment that doesn't protect them.

2. It must fit you. Equipment that doesn't fit won't give you enough protection.

3. It must be comfortable. Equipment that sits in your locker because it doesn't fit, or is too bulky or heavy isn't doing anything for your health and safety on the job.

4. You must know how to use the equipment, when to use it, and why—through proper training and instruction.

5. The equipment must be taken care of and stored properly.

Personal protective equipment can range all the way from complete clothing outfits to devices designed to protect only certain parts of your body.

Protective clothing may include overalls, aprons, smocks, pants, hoods, or a combination of them. The main idea is to keep harmful substances from getting on your skin or penetrating it. The particular articles used will depend on the point of possible contact—face, arms, hands, legs and so on. Some jobs may require complete head-to-toe coverings.

In some cases, you may have to use two lockers—one for the protective clothing you wear on the job, and the other for your street clothes. This will eliminate the risk of carrying home toxic substances. Workers' families have become ill from poisons brought home on work clothes.

Whenever there is a danger of head injuries caused by falling or flying objects, hard hats are required by OSHA regulations. A bunch of nonsense, you say? Government studies show that more than 80 percent of workers who sufffered head injuries were not wearing hard hats.

Eye injuries disable about 130,000 workers on the job each year. Your eyes—your most precious tools—are exposed to a wide range of dangers: flying particles, chemical splashes, irritating dusts and fumes. Depending on the job, eye protection can be anything from simple goggles to welding helmets. In all cases where there is danger from flying particles, the glasses should be shatter-proof. If you need corrective lenses, they must be fitted by a professional.

Respirators control exposure to contaminated air or, in other situations, supply air where there is not enough. Among all protective equipment, respirators require the most careful choosing, fitting and use. You must know what the substance is that you are being protected from, how concentrated it is, how dangerous it is, and how long you're going to be exposed. If your's doesn't fit, it isn't working for you. Don't settle for anything that isn't right. There's no room for "next best" when the very air you breathe is the problem.

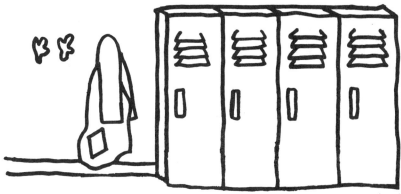

If noise can't be reduced at the source, ear muffs or plugs are better than nothing. Choose the type that's most comfortable for you and that will give you the necessary protection. Cotton in the ears, incidentally, does not protect you from dangerous noise levels.

Personal protection on the job, ideally, should begin at the source of the hazard by eliminating the dangers through mechanical and engineering changes, cutting down the time you may be exposed, and so on. Until then, your best bet is personal protective equipment. Get to know it. Use it. Take care of it. It can help take care of you.

The Right Type of Respirator

Most industrial chemicals enter the body by inhalation. They are in the air as dusts, mists, gases, fumes or vapors. Respirators put a barrier between these hazards suspended in the air we breathe and our lungs. There are two major classes of respirators:

1. *Air purifying.* These clean the air that is inhaled.
2. *Air supplying.* These provide workers with their own supply of air or oxygen.

There are four types of air purifying respirators: The mechanical filter type cleans the air of dust and fumes by trapping them in a bed of fibers. The chemical cartridge kind cleans the air of vapors by absorbing them into some material such as charcoal. These are used when the worker is exposed to solvents or chemicals with a high vapor pressure. A combination respirator protects against dusts, vapors, fumes and/or mists. Gas mask respirators may either trap gas or use chemicals to change the gas to a non-toxic form.

There are three basic types of air supplying respirators. They differ in the source of the clean air they supply.

In the hose mask type, the free end of a hose runs from the worker's mask to an area that is free of contamination. The airline type supplies the worker with air by attaching the free end of the hose to a stationary compressed air source. The third type—called supplied air—provides air from tanks carried by the worker.

There are some cautions you should know about if you use either of the two types of respirators. The air purifiers should NOT be used when there is exposure to: cancer causing substances; unknown chemicals; unknown concentration of chemicals; chemicals that are immediately dangerous to life or health; chemicals that produce their toxic effects below the level where you can smell them.

The air purifying type also should not be used in areas where the oxygen concentration is too low to support life. This means less than 19 percent by volume. Air purifiers also have a limited lifetime. If you smell something coming through your respirator, it is no longer effective. Gas mask canisters should have color indicators, visible to the wearer, that indicate when a canister is no longer providing protection.

If your work takes you into an area where the air is immediately dangerous to life and health, only supplied air respirators can be used. Remember, your airline is your life line. Air hoses can be cut, leaving you without protection.

There are also limitations to the use of respirators. These devices are designed to protect only against specific types of substances, and within certain ranges of concentration. It is important for you to know what chemical or toxic substance you are working with so you can use the correct respirator designed for that particular situation.

The thin seal of a respirator can break when the wearer is talking or moving quickly. If this happens, the toxic substance can enter through the facepiece. Some workers have a hard time getting a good facepiece seal due to facial hair or because the facepiece never really fit.

The Occupational Safety and Health Administration (OSHA) requires that all workers whose jobs require them to wear a respirator be test fitted. There are two ways to do this and make sure the wearer has a good seal between the respirator and the face:

1. In "quantitative" testing, the worker goes into a closed booth while wearing a respirator. A test solution is placed in the booth and a machine measures the concentration of the solution both inside the respirator and outside it in the booth. By comparing these two readings, any leakage can be determined.

2. In "qualitative" testing, some kind of test substance—irritant smoke or banana oil—is passed three inches from the respirator the worker is wearing. If the wearer can smell the smoke or oil, the respirator does not fit.

Qualitative testing gives a simple "yes" or "no" about whether a facepiece fits. It takes the more precise quantitative test to show the degree of fitting—how well the respirator is doing its job.

Air Sampling—Why and How?

The sense of smell has remarkable capabilities. The aroma of sizzling bacon and fresh-perked coffee can often rouse the groggiest sleepyhead. Certain fragrances have been used for romantic turn-ons since antiquity. And body odor has wafted a multibillion-dollar industry of daintiness.

But when it comes to warning you of possibly dangerous air contamination in the workplace, your nose and sense of smell are not so capable. Hazardous airborne contaminants may be masked by other odors. Some life-threatening contaminants have no smell at all—carbon monoxide, for example.

To sniff out these dangers before they have a chance to harm you, various sophisticated air sampling devices and techniques have been developed. In the hands of a professional industrial hygienist, these devices can provide such information as:

- Whether a contaminant is present;
- How much of it is in the air, and whether the level is within the limits set up to protect your health;
- Where the contamination probably is coming from.

Sampling also is useful for testing the effectiveness of engineering controls, such as a local ventilation system or an enclosure of an operation. These measurements also can tell whether the safety measures in place are adequate, or whether there are enough of them, or whether they're in the right place and so on.

Sampling can be particularly important when changes are made in a production process that could have the potential for generating new hazardous substances.

There are several ways of sampling. "Grab sampling," as the name implies, is done periodically during a shift at particular times and at a particular place during a production cycle. By analyzing these samples, the industrial hygienist can chart the changes, if any, during the cycle.

Grab samples are useful in a number of ways. They can measure ceiling levels—that is, the level a worker must not be exposed to regardless of the shortness of the exposure time. This type of sampling also is used to measure levels of exposure that can be tolerated for short, specified intervals. Grab samples also are useful in determining which part of the work process is causing the contamination so that engineering controls can be designed and put in place.

Unlike this kind of spot check, "integrated sampling" measures a worker's exposure over an extended time, usually the entire shift. Integrated sampling also differs from grab sampling in that it can provide a composite of the worker's exposure in the various areas of the workplace where he or she might go.

In order to do this, a small sampling device is often worn by the worker. These detectors may be passive; that is, they may have no mechanical parts and collect the samples simply by exposure to the air. Other types of integrated sampling devices use a pump to pull the contaminated air through a collection medium. In both cases, the devices are usually attached to the lapels or collar of the worker's clothing so that they will measure as closely as possible the contamination in the worker's immediate breathing space.

It is part of the industrial hygienist's job to determine which type of air sampling is appropriate. The decision may be based on a preliminary study of the operation, including the substances used, the product that is being made, and the possible by-products the process may give off.

The industrial hygienist also will consider other factors beside the kinds of contaminants that may be encountered. For example, sampling may be extended over a long enough period of time to take into account the various intensities that a worker may be exposed to during the production cycle. A sample taken over a short period may not produce results which represent the overall average of exposure.

Another factor that must be considered is that airborne contaminants may be concentrated in pockets instead of being distributed uniformly throughout the work area. Particular matter larger than that which can be normally breathed tend to settle quickly on workplace surfaces. In such cases, "wipe samples" are often used to estimate past exposure. PCB, lead, and regulated carcinogens are often collected by wipe sampling.

Workplace Design

"Ergonomics" is a funny looking word with a serious meaning for your comfort and health. In everyday language, the word simply means making jobs fit people—not people fit jobs. It comes from the Greek "ergon" (work) and "nomos" (law).

A lot of aches and pains, sprains and strains, could be eliminated if workplace design followed the principles of ergonomics. A well-designed workplace takes into acount the varying sizes and strengths of the entire workforce, including the handicapped. Here are a few ideas from just one part of ergonomics—"biomechanics"—dealing mostly with the way you use (or misuse) your arms, legs and back.

Tools and equipment should be designed so that your hands and wrists are in the same position as if they were hanging relaxed at your side. If the tool, or the position you are required to use it in, bends your wrists, that's bad design.

Where possible, jobs should be designed so that the arms don't have to be raised above shoulder height on a regular basis. Good design tries to follow two principles:

- Keep your arms low,
- Keep your elbows close to your body.

Holding the muscles tense in a fixed position is more tiring than using moving muscles. The movement allows the muscles to relax momentarily. An example of this "dynamic" versus "static" work would be holding a board steady with one hand while you sawed with the other. In general, static work should be designed out by using tools or clamping devices instead of holding by hand.

Work tasks should be designed to take the best mechanical advantage of the muscles used. This avoids overloading the muscles. For instance, where jobs require arm strength, the exertion should be in and out, not across the body.

Back injuries are one of the leading—if not *the* leading— causes of job-related disabilities. And a major share of the blame lies with workplace design that makes people work with a bent spine. Jobs should be designed to allow workers to work with their backs straight.

Improper lifting probably causes as much back misery as any single cause. Remember: keep the back straight and lift with the legs, keeping the load as close to the body as possible. Don't twist or turn the spine while carrying the load.

Standing still for too long can put excessive stress on the spine and back muscles, causing pain and even permanent damage to body tissue. A foot rest—like the old saloon "brass rail"—lessens stress on the back. You should change leg position often.

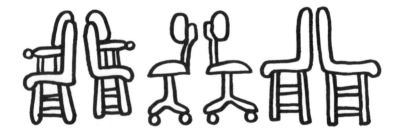

Poorly designed or mismatched chairs and work benches can cause fatigue and circulation problems, especially at such critical points as the knees and waist. Proper height of the work surface depends on the nature of the work. Precision work, where you have to see closely, should be high; low if the work requires heavy manipulation, pressure or lifting.

The United Automobile, Aerospace and Agricultural Implement Workers (UAW) has published a booklet containing an action plan to help correct poor workplace design. Among the steps suggested are:

- Survey the workforce to find out who has symptoms of sprains and strains, and get workers' ideas about how to correct problems;
- Document medical problems by reviewing OSHA injury records, workers' compensation records, sickness and accident records, and visits to the company medical department;
- Evaluate all jobs and operations for poor set-up and design;
- Establish a system of communications so that all affected parties—management, engineers, union representatives, skilled trades and production workers—have input into decisions;
- Set up priorities and a systematic method of correcting problems.

Workers are not interchangeable parts you can reach in a bin for. They are flesh and blood, old and young, short and tall, weak and strong, male and female, All of these variables have to be taken into account in good job and workplace design.

Safety and Health in Contracts

Despite solid gains for workplace safety and health over the years through collective bargaining, there's still too much truth to the old line that work is an occupational hazard.

Potentially hazardous chemicals and other substances are introduced at an astonishing rate throughout industry in our increasingly technological society. New machines and new processes come on line without any clear vision as to their long-range consequences for workers' safety and health. In too many cases, the human body is the proving ground. We are obliged to mend people—not change the machines that are the real culprits.

The long latency period of some potentially toxic substances—the hidden dangers that don't show up for many years—complicates efforts to ensure that workers won't pay the price of progress with ill health and disability far down the road.

Collective bargaining to nail down safety and health guarantees in union contracts remains the primary protection for workers. Some mossback managements may still resist this. They cling to the outdated notion that safety and health are solely a "management prerogative."

Some employers fear they will lose control over decisions affecting work processes and methods, or the choice of materials and equipment. Finally, they bring up the old bugaboo that engineering controls to reduce or eliminate hazards would cost too much.

Not all employers are like this, of course. Some enlightened companies have been persuaded that effective safety and health measures reduce the cost of workers' compensation and boost morale and productivity.

It is impossible in a short space to list all the ingredients of good contract language regarding safety and health. There are too many different circumstances to cover with a single, all-purpose checklist. But there are some general guidelines. Two bedrock positions for negotiations are:

1. *Legal.* Safety and health are mandatory subjects for collective bargaining. That was established in 1966 by the National Labor Relations Board (NLRB) in the Gulf Power Co. case. That decision knocked the props from under the old "management prerogative" smokescreen. The Occupational Safety and Health Act of 1970, although originally based on "voluntary compliance," mandates that all workplaces be safe and healthful environments.

2. *Philosophical.* Negotiators are on sound ground when they insist from the beginning that human life cannot be reduced to cost terms. Workers' safety and health are not negotiable; trade-offs are not acceptable.

Next, a tightly written general duty clause is essential. This clause assures you that your employer is committed to providing a safe and healthful workplace, and will obey all local, state and federal laws and regulations with regard to health and safety. This clause lets you file a grievance over violations without having to call in an inspector.

The language must be specific. Many otherwise good contracts have been watered down by language such as: "The employer shall continue to make reasonable provisions for the safety and health of employees during the hours of employment." Watch out for wishy-washy words like "reasonable." A company's "reasonable" policy may be a worker's poison.

Contract clauses also should cover in detail such broad areas as: duties of the company, employee rights, recognition of the union's safety and health committee, and access to information. Here are a few specific suggestions from a workers' guide published by the AFL-CIO Food and Allied Service Trades Department:

• Company responsibilities: Regular medical examinations to diagnose and monitor occupational diseases by the worker's own doctor at company expense; protective equipment and clothing; safety education and training; warning signs to indicate hazardous conditions; clean and sanitary rest, locker, shower, lunch and break rooms.
• Workers' rights: Refusal of hazardous work; transfer to another position if seriously impaired by a work-related illness or injury; lost time pay for an industrial injury; regular pay for time spent on an OSHA

inspection, and freedom from company reprisals for exercising your legal rights.

- Safety and health committee rights: Recognition by the company; compensation at regular rates for members' time spent on safety and health issues (including committee meetings); plant surveys for hazards; accident investigations; right to use testing and monitoring equipment.
- Information: Hazardous materials used, their chemical compounds and appropriate protective measures; results of company-paid medical exams; access to injury, illness and exposure records.

How Records Track Killer Risks

From the day we're born to the day we die, important times in the lives of most of us are written down by somebody and filed, or stored in a computer's memory. Remember the long questionnaires you had to fill out when you applied for a job and went to work? Did you wonder: "Why do I have to fill out all these forms?" One good answer: Those records can be important to your health and the health of your co-workers.

Such records—yours and all those of others in your line of work—make up one of the basic tools used in epidemiological studies of occupational hazards. (The word "epidemiology" comes from "epidemic"—affecting a lot of people at the same time in a locality—and "-logy"—the body of knowledge about a subject.)

Taken together, all these individual pieces of information give the epidemiologist—a sort of medical detective—an overall picture of a particular work group, including age, sex, race, length of employment and so on. In studying hazardous exposures, it's better to use a group like this rather than the general public because:

- The occupational group is better defined and more accessible for follow-up.
- The exposure generally is uniform or similar.
- The exposure is usually at a higher concentration than that experienced by the general population.

Now, suppose an epidemiologist wants to find out the mortality risk of Substance X to a particular group of exposed workers. First, a time frame is set up—say from January 1, 1949, to the end of 1980. The study group, or cohort, will consist of everybody who ever worked at the plant or industry during that span of time. The study must cover an extended interval to produce reliable data because some substances (like asbestos) may take a long time to produce ill effects.

Then, by studying the death rate for the workers and comparing this rate with the rate of deaths among a control group of the same characteristics, the epidemiologist can begin to get some idea about the deadly effects of Substance X on exposed workers. Not all studies are based on death rates. Some measure the incidence of disease.

Of course, it's not as simple as that. Obviously, there are many variations in the makeup of the study group. Given the long time span, some workers may have died; others have worked for varying lengths of time in that particular plant or industry; still others simply have been lost for follow-up. So all the people don't contribute equally to the "population at risk" for statistical purposes.

To get around this, researchers use the concept of "person-years." Each employee is followed from the date of the study, or the first date of employment (or exposure) to the date of death (if that has occurred). Each of these individuals is also classified by age, sex and race.

Now the data is more finely focused. Age-sex-race-cause-specific mortality rates can be compared to similar data compiled on a national basis. If there are more deaths than should be expected for a given number of person-years with similar age, sex and race characteristics, then Substance X poses a problem.

This is a greatly oversimplified example of how these medical detectives work to gauge occupational hazards. There are many more leads to follow, especially in tracking down employees who have left the particular study group. This involves getting many more records—vital status information (living or dead), personnel files, seniority lists, Social Security, even drivers' licenses, and change-of-address information from the postal service.

All this may not make you enjoy filling out forms. But at least you know it's not to satisfy some nosy person's curiosity. Over the years, epidemiology can make you and your workplace healthier.

Keeping Personal Health Records

"Sure, I suspect a lot of the stuff that goes on around here is bad for my health, but what can I do?"

"Yeah, I know guys who have got sick or hurt on this job, but that's for the boss to worry about."

"Okay, the place I work is hot and stinks. What's the union health and safety committee doing about it?"

164

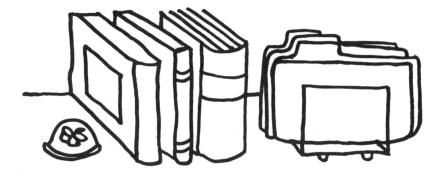

Does that kind of talk sound familiar? Do you recognize yourself? You as an individual can help yourself, your fellow workers and your union by getting more involved in what your job and the place you work are doing to your health. The "let-George-do-it" attitude makes it harder and slower to clean up health hazards around the workplace. So, how do you start?

Keep a pocket notebook or log. Put down all accidents, injuries and illnesses that occur. Update your log with every new job or process you work with.

Your own health notebook can be coordinated with the experiences of others in your place of work. The overall picture can help to provide the documentation to correct unhealthy conditions and practices.

Extensive evidence is generally needed to prove a link between health problems and on-the-job exposure to hazardous substances. That is why your own records, combined with those of others in your group, are important parts in developing an effective, long-range strategy for eliminating work hazards.

Workers can conduct their own surveys of plants and the departments they work in. They should take note of chemicals, dust, fumes, gases, noise and ventilation. Most individuals and local unions don't have the equipment to actually monitor exposure levels. Even so, a walk-through survey of conditions, machines, processes, storage and the like is an important step in cleaning up and maintaining the workplace.

Naturally, the employer is the best source of information about what chemicals are used, the manufacturing processes, etc. But, in most cases, the management is not required to provide employees with this information. You and your union may have to fight for this over the bargaining table and through legislation.

But there is one notable exception to this possible problem of getting information. Since 1980, an Occupational Safety and Health Administration (OSHA) standard has been in effect that grants workers access to certain vital records. Upon written request to the employer, you, or a representative designated by you, must be provided with:

- Medical records and any analysis using these records,
- Exposure records and any analysis using these exposure records.

The exposure information should include records of workplace monitoring, biological monitoring, material safety data sheets, and a list of all toxic substances or harmful physical agents used in the workplace.

Many companies keep files on previous employment, periodic medical exams, and work-related injuries and illnesses. Some are more complete and helpful than others, depending on the quality of each company's medical program. The records you keep yourself about your own experiences, combined with similar individual records of people you work with, can often supplement company records in important ways.

Union locals or health and safety committees should keep their own files on members. These files should include not only the personally kept records and those from the employer, but also worker complaints, grievances, and minutes of meetings with management, government officials and others. Inactive files should be kept as long as possible because many health problems—reproductive effects, or the consequences of asbestos exposure, for example—may not show up until years after the initial exposure.

If you suspect a problem, you should contact your union, the National Institute for Occupational Safety and Health, or other organizations or individuals you trust to help you.

What to Do About Hazards

Do you sometimes wonder about the hazards to your health and safety from some of the chemicals or other materials you work with? Many workers do worry about this—and with good cause.

Do you know how to find out what's in these products? What they might do to you? How you can protect yourself?

One way is to ask your employer for the information supplied by the manufacturer. If this doesn't work, why not go right to "the horse's mouth"—the manufacturer himself?

If you don't know the name of a specific individual or department, address your letter to "Consumer Information" in care of the company that makes the products. Your letter might follow this form, suggested by the Workers Health Center in Lidcombe, Australia. (The names, of course, are fictitious.)

Dear Sir/Madam:

I am writing to ask if you would supply me with information about the possible health hazards of one (some) of your products:

SLUDGO XP1

SOLVOTRIX X4

I am (shop steward/safety representative/union secretary) at CHE-MOTRIX CO. and I (my members) use SLUDGO and SOLVOTRIX at work. I would like information on:

1. Composition. What are the chemical ingredients of SLUDGO and SOLVOTRIX; the chemical formula of each, and the rough proportion in which they are mixed?

2. Impurities. What impurities could there be in the finished product?

3. Harmful effects. What harmful effects are these substances known or suspected to cause in humans? What harmful effects have been found in animals? Please include reports of both short- and long-term tests on these substances.

4. Have there been any tests of carcinogenicity, such as the AMES test, or other long-term effects/illnesses?

5. Routes of entry. With exposure, what are the likely routes of entry into the body: inhalation, swallowing, skin absorption, eye contact, etc?

6. Safe levels. At what concentration or dose, and what period of exposure, were any ill effects observed?

7. Other safety hazards. What other health or safety hazards might arise from using these substances, such as fire, explosion?

8. Control methods. What precautions should be taken when working with or near SLUDGO and SOLVOTRIX; for example, ventilation, protective clothing, goggles and the like?

9. What threshold limit value (TLV) or other control limit do you recommend for these substances?

10. Clean up. If a chemical spills or leaks out, what precautions should be taken in the clean-up? Is there a disposal method to avoid environmental pollution?

11. Over-exposure/first aid. What symptoms indicate that over-exposure has occurred, and what first aid measures should be taken?

Your cooperation in helping to clear up these points will be appreciated. I look forward to hearing from you.

Sincerely,

Your union's health and safety committee, or some other designated group or individual, already may have much of this sort of information, especially on some of the older, better known products. But new materials with different ingredients are introduced into the workplace all the time. It is to your advantage to know as much about them as possible. If you can't get satisfaction from your employer, write directly to the source.

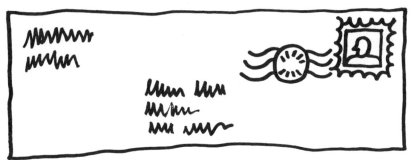

Union Safety and Health Committees

A Safety and Health Committee—if it's on the ball—can be a strong asset for a union.

"Oh yeah? Like what?" skeptical members might ask. These doubting Thomases (and Thomasinas) probably believe the old joke about a giraffe being a horse put together by a committee. But, in truth, a Safety and Health Committee has many opportunities to do a good job for you and your union.

If your union already has such a committee, here is a checklist of some things it can be doing. If your union is thinking about forming such a committee, the same list can be used to set some goals. The list is adapted from one prepared by the American Federation of State, County and Municipal Employees (AFSCME). The main functions of the committee should include:

- Making frequent plant safety tours, investigating serious safety violations and accidents, and filing and following up on OSHA complaints;
- Assisting other local committees on grievances, contract language on safety, and safety training;
- Taking part in safety training provided by the AFL-CIO, individual unions, various universities, and OSHA;
- Keeping informed on OSHA and state laws and policies, and going to bat and lobbying for safety and health legislation at all levels of government;
- Reviewing the employer's use of toxic materials, hazardous machinery and equipment, as well as remodeling or construction that may cause safety and health problems.

A good Safety and Health Committee also can train its members in the use of basic industrial hygiene instruments. These should include a sound-level meter, Botsball heat-stress thermometer, gas and vapor detector, and velometer (for ventilation). It's a good idea to buy a basic instrument kit for the local.

The local union's library should include copies of safety codes and regulations, as well as training materials, in safety, industrial hygiene, and occupational diseases.

There are a couple of organizational "do's" and "don'ts" suggested by the State, County and Municipal Employees: DO make the Safety and Health Committee a standing committee of the union local. DON'T set it up to compete with the Grievance/Bargaining Committee. It should be set up, instead, to assist that committee.

AFSCME hangs out a red warning flag on "joint safety committees" with the employer. Such "consultative" devices are often used by management, the public employees union explains, "to avoid bargaining with the union on an equal basis over safety matters."

The employer can argue, often convincingly, that safety and health are "cooperative" goals of both the union and management. The existence of a joint committee also gives management "good faith" credit with OSHA. In most cases, however, it probably isn't a good idea for a union to participate in a joint committee unless it has equal control and is already operating from a strong union committee.

Another point to remember: The union and the employer often have conflicting interests when it comes to safety matters. Each side looks from a different viewpoint on such issues as the cost of safety improvements, acting on OSHA complaints, or identifying occupational diseases.

In evaluating a joint committee, the union should ask:

- Do the union and the employer have an equal number of members?
- Does the union have the sole right to appoint its representatives?
- Do the positions of chairperson and secretary rotate between the two parties?
- Who makes up the agenda and approves the minutes?
- Is there a neutral procedure for breaking tie votes?
- Does the committee have access to all company data on monitoring, toxic materials, relative costs of safety materials, relative costs of safety improvements, workers' compensation records?

These are hard-headed, but sensible, questions. They are not intended to throw cold water on the idea of shared concerns and responsibilities; certainly not on the idea of a union Safety and Health Committee. But, as stated in the beginning, to make the idea work, you've got to keep your eye on the ball. Otherwise, you might end up with a giraffe instead of a workhorse.

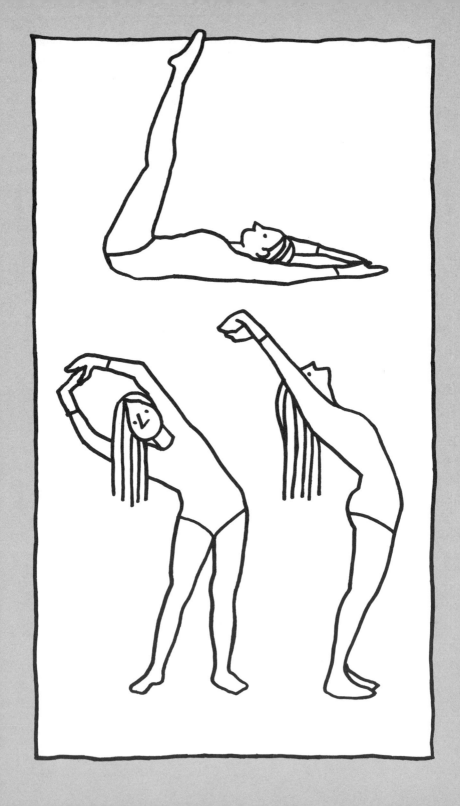

7 Enhancing Workers' Health

Live Right—and Live Longer

The total cost of health care in the United States is well over $300 billion a year—more than $1,300 for every man, woman and child. From each of those dollars, about 97 cents goes to treat sickness. A paltry 3 cents is spent on promoting "wellness." Does that kind of split seem cockeyed? It does to growing numbers of Americans. So, the idea is beginning to sink in that it's better—cheaper and more fun—to stay well than it is to pay for being sick. One approach to putting this idea into practice is something called "prospective medicine."

About 20 years ago, Dr. Lewis C. Robbins and Dr. Jack Hall developed the concept at the Methodist Hospital of Indiana in Indianapolis. They figured that it is better to deal with a prospective disease when a known cause is evident (like smoking), or when you reach a certain age, or enter an environment that may be risky for you, than at a later time. If you wait until the symptoms of disease show up—whether you notice them or they are detected by laboratory tests or physical examination—it is often too late to cure the problem.

A key tool in the practice of prospective medicine is the Health Hazard Appraisal. This is a sort of "health bank balance." It tells you what chances you are taking with your life, and how you can improve your odds of surviving the next 10 years.

In a pamphlet on Health Hazard Appraisal she wrote for the Public Affairs Committee, Lydia Ratcliff started off with a list of questions. They are similar to what you might be asked in an appraisal:

- Are you 15 percent (or more) overweight?
- Do you eat beef, lamb or pork one or more times a day?
- Do you exercise only rarely?
- Do you smoke a pack or more of cigarettes a day?
- Do you take tranquilizers or pills—in increasing amounts—to pep up, to calm you down, or to help you sleep?
- Do you take chances while driving a car?

Let's say you are a young American adult and you answered "yes" to all the questions. Your chances of living to age 50 are about 50-50.

Suppose you answered "yes" to only three. You still may be paying 10 years out of the lifespan you might otherwise look forward to because of the way you're living.

But there's a brighter side to this health bank balance idea. Like your regular savings account, you can make deposits as well as withdrawals. You probably can "buy back" some of those years you have been spending if you make certain changes now.

This idea was tested in a California study which suggested seven healthy lifestyle practices:

1. Get seven to eight hours of sleep a night.
2. Eat breakfast.
3. Eat regularly, and avoid between-meal snacks.
4. Keep normal weight in relation to height.
5. Refrain from smoking.
6. Exercise regularly.
7. Drink very moderately.

The results of the California study showed that men and women who followed six of the seven recommendations had significantly higher life expectancies than people who followed fewer than four. Men could expect to live 11 years longer; women, 7 years longer.

Of course, there are some risk factors that can't be reduced. You can't do much about any negative prospects associated with your actual age, sex, family history of a disease, race or ethnic background—all of which can play a part in how healthy you are and how long you can expect to live.

Dr. John Hanlon, former assistant surgeon general of the U.S. Public Health Service, put it in sporting terms: "Good odds alone do not guarantee [a win], but the reality is that the better the odds, based on sound information, the better the chance of winning."

Ask your doctor, local health organization or union representative about the Health Hazard Appraisal. Find out who's giving them in your locality, and how much they cost. It's well worth looking into. In the biggest game of all—your life—you may be able to tilt the odds in your favor—if you're willing.

Common Sense—Guide to Good Diet

Food is the fuel that keeps your body's machinery working. Diet, broadly speaking, is simply how you manage the fueling process. Like most high-performance engines, your body requires a blended fuel. You put this together by using ingredients from four basic food groups: 1. Breads and cereals. 2. Protein foods. 3. Milk and milk products. 4. Fruits and vegetables. How well you do this determines your diet—good or bad— and, to a large extent, how well you function as a healthy machine.

Breads, pasta and cereal grains contribute several B vitamins and iron. These are essential for growth and all major body functions. The foods may be either whole grain or enriched, but whole grains contain more vitamins and minerals. B vitamins and iron are also found in red meat, liver, peas and beans. Other sources of iron are leafy green vegetables and dried fruits such as raisins.

Protein foods help build blood and tissues like skin, hair and muscles. Generally, the most complete proteins are found in meat, fish, milk, cheese and eggs. It is also possible to get complete protein by eating only vegetable protein if you know the right combination to use with the protein from grain sources. In addition to grains, vegetarian protein is also found in peas, beans, seeds and nuts.

However, it is easier to meet the body's need for protein by including in the diet some animal sources along with the vegetables and grain. The amount from animal sources need not be large. For example, a glass of milk along with the right combination of vegetables and grain may supply enough protein.

Among other things, milk and milk products contribute calcium and riboflavin. These are important for the hardness of teeth and bones. They also help your heart, muscles and nerve tissue work properly, and are needed for blood coagulation during bleeding.

Calcium in fair amounts is found in all hard cheeses such as cheddars, Swiss and Jack. Calcium is also found in soybean cake (tofu), calcium treated tortillas, and dark leafy vegetables such as kale, mustard greens and spinach. But this vegetable source of calcium sometimes has a drawback since the calcium may be found in combination with oxalic acid. This chemical makes the calcium less available to your body. Unless you eat a large amount of vegetables, or are allergic to milk, your diet should include some milk products.

The fourth food group—fruits and vegetables—probably offers the widest variety of good nutrients. Unfortunately, it is the one source many Americans tend to slight. This is too bad because these foods are particularly important sources of vitamins A and C. Besides, they provide a wide range of flavors and eye appeal for the diet.

You need vitamin A to maintain good night vision, to promote bone growth, and to help your body resist infection. While vitamin A is found only in foods of animal origin, a substance called carotene—contained in leafy green vegetables and in many yellow fruits and vegetables—can be changed to vitamin A in the body. Vitamin A is found in large amounts

173

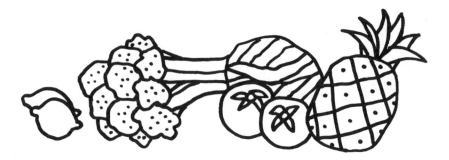

in liver and in smaller amounts in eggs, milk, butter and margarine.

Vitamin C is probably the best known of the vitamins. It is important for healthy bones, teeth and gums, and for the healing of wounds. All citrus fruits and juices, as well as cantaloupes, strawberries and green peppers, are good sources of vitamin C. You can get a fair amount of vitamin C from other fruits and vegetables.

How you prepare foods can affect their nutritional value. Many vitamins and minerals can be lost in cooking. You can cut this loss by washing and cooking foods as quickly as possible. Don't clean vegetables by soaking. And when you cook them, add only a little water.

Snacks, such as candy and soft drinks, were not included in the four basic food groups for good reasons. They don't offer much nutritionally, and they can have some bad effects if indulged in to excess. We eat too much sugar—about 125 pounds per person per year. About 20 percent of our calories comes from sugar. Many nutritionists think we should be getting less than 10 percent from that source.

Besides causing tooth decay, sugar is also linked to diabetes and hypoglycemia (low blood sugar). Eating too much sugar also interferes with your body's ability to absorb calcium, and may result in vitamin B deficiency.

Common sense is still the best rule for good food habits. Eat something from each of the four basic food groups every day, but don't go overboard. Keep your weight normal. Eat less salt. (Studies indicate a relationship between salt and high blood pressure.) If you drink, and you're overweight, remember those alcoholic beverages are loaded with calories and have virtually no nutritional value.

The Value of Worthwhile Work

What's the first thing that comes to mind when you see or hear the words, "work and health"? A lot of people, probably most, think of the bad effects of work on health: The toxic fumes you might breathe on the job. The caustics that can splash on your skin or into your eyes. The backaches from improper lifting. The unseen and unfelt ill effects of radiation, and so on and on.

But let's look at another side of "work and health"—the bad effects of "un-work" brought on by unemployment or retirement. Can the lack of work also harm your health? Yes, indeed!

Enforced idleness—for whatever reason—among people who are willing and able to work can skew the way we feel about ourselves and others, generally in negative ways. These twisted, negative feelings are especially damaging to our mental health, which plays such an important role in determining our physical wellbeing.

As far back as the Great Depression of the 1930s, for example, studies found that loss of work produced cynicism, loss of self-confidence, resentment, hostility, feelings of helplessness and isolation. Obviously, these negative feelings are not a good foundation for physical and mental health.

Similar findings showed up again a few years ago in a government study on "Work in America." In this study, the authors wrote: "It is clear from recent research that work plays a crucial and perhaps unparalleled psychological role in the formation of self-esteem, identity and a sense of order." More recently, Dr. Harvey Brenner, a sociologist at Johns Hopkins University, found that an increase in the rate of unemployment was reflected to some degree in the rise in the death rate.

Still another example: In a 15-year study of the aging process, what do you suppose Erdman Palmore of Duke University's sociology department found was the strongest factor in predicting longevity? Work satisfaction. And the second best indicator? Overall "happiness."

These two factors—satisfying work and happiness—were better at predicting how long people would live than a rating of their chances by a physician who looked only at the physical functioning of their bodies.

Undoubtedly, there are other factors that are important in extending life—diet, exercise, medical care, and the kind of genes we inherit. But research indicates that those factors may account for only about 25 percent of the risk factors in heart disease, the major cause of death.

This raises an interesting question: What about that unexplained 75 percent of risk factors? Although research has not led to conclusive answers, it appears that the way we see our role as workers, and our working conditions and other social factors, may contribute heavily to our physical and mental health.

Loss of self-esteem and identity are not just reserved for people out of work. The feeling of being without roots or a purpose in life can also affect workers who are still on the job; who may, indeed, have been on the job for years.

175

Their problem may be summed up in the question they may secretly ask themselves: "Does what I do really matter?" This feeling about ourselves—that we *do* count for something—plays a vital part in our health. We can't pinpoint it as accurately as we can spot a telltale medical problem, but it is there just as surely as the breath of life itself.

Thomas R. Donahue, secretary-treasurer of the AFL-CIO, said it well in the *American Federationist* magazine:

It is a provable fact—and not a "bleeding heart" philosophical speculation—that workers produce more when they have a sense of creative involvement in their work, when they feel that what they do is relevant, that it serves a useful purpose, and that their work is appreciated. Most important of all, workers respond positively to the sense of dignity and respect gained from the work they do. . . .

Where worker participation and decision-making involving their work has been high, studies have shown a corresponding drop in absenteeism, turnover, filing of grievances, and even trips to the employee health center.

Albert Camus, the French novelist, summed it up: "Without work, all life goes rotten. But when work is soulless, life stifles and dies."

The Importance of Medical Check-ups

Medical check-ups mean different things to different people:

"Every time I go in for my regular physical I start shaking like a leaf."

"Why bother? I feel okay."

"My doctor orders all these lab tests and I don't know any more afterward than I did before."

Scared? Devil-may-care? Puzzled? Let's try to take some of the mystery out of this subject of medical check-ups. The more you understand, the better partner you can become with your doctor in caring for your health.

First of all, a medical exam—the kind of check-up you should have at regular intervals—is not a diagnosis. By itself, a test won't tell you or your doctor what's wrong with you if you are having a problem. What the results can do—if they fall outside a "normal" range, for example—is to provide clues. These clues can tell your doctor where to look for possible trouble, and what to look for. It's the interpretation, not the tests themselves, that counts.

Take blood tests. A few drops of blood from a single pin-prick can provide a complete blood-cell count. The red cells carry oxygen to body tissues. A low count may indicate anemia, possibly as a result of hidden blood loss or excessive menstrual bleeding. An excess of red blood cells may indicate illness.

White cells make up the SWAT team of the blood, ready to battle invaders. If the white cell count is excessive, it may mean an infection, leukemia or allergy. A low count could indicate radiation or exposure to toxic chemicals.

In addition to the cell count, blood also can be analyzed for various chemical substances. There are enzymes from the liver and muscles, alkaline phosphates from liver or bone, blood urea nitrogen (a measure of kidney function), uric acid (a possible indicator of gout), sodium, potassium and chloride, among others.

Another substance found in the blood is cholesterol, a waxy alcohol. This material can become part of the deposits that clog arteries. Studies have linked high levels of serum cholesterol to increased risk of heart disease. (Serum is the pale yellowish liquid that separates from blood when it clots.)

Cholesterol is a two-faced substance. While the total amount is important, perhaps even more significant are the fractions that make up the whole. There is the part known as HDL, which stands for high-density lipoprotein cholesterol. This type is believed to help protect against heart disease. Then there are LDL and VLDL, for low- and very-low-density lipoprotein cholesterol. Both of these are suspected of contributing to heart disease.

The relative distribution of these types is a clue your doctor will be looking for. If your blood test shows a high total cholesterol count and a low level of the high-density lipoprotein type, for example, your doctor may suggest cutting down of fats and cholesterol, getting more exercise and losing weight, if you're on the heavy side.

Too much sugar in the blood (or urine) can be a clue to a diabetic condition—present or about about to develop—as well as other health problems.

Low-blood sugar, or hypoglycemia, can be properly diagnosed after a dramatic drop in sugar at the same time the patient feels such symptoms as weakness, headache or nausea.

Here are three things you can do to make your regular medical check-ups more useful:

1. Ask your doctor to explain things you don't understand.
2. Tell your doctor about anything unusual in your current way of living that could affect the tests—prescription and over-the-counter drugs you may be taking (even aspirin, vitamins and birth control pills), alcohol, lack of sleep, stress, fear or anxiety.
3. Keep a record of important tests and put down the dates.

As a worker, you know about preventive maintenance. Take care of things while they're still working, not after they break down. Think about your regular check-ups in the same way—even though you feel great.

Doctor and Patient Communication

It's one of the most persistent and widespread medical complaints. It's common among both men and women of all ages, in all walks of life. Its symptoms are a feeling of general irritation, often accompanied by heat under the collar. Its name: "Misunderstandingitis"—an inflammation in the doctor-patient relationship. It can lead to poorer health care for you.

If you've got this complaint, what can you do to help heal the breach?

The root of the problem is a breakdown in communication. Prepare yourself in advance for a visit to the doctor. Know the main reason you're going and tell the doctor—flat out! Don't beat around the bush.

You'd be surprised at how many patients come into the office and don't mention the main thing that's troubling them, probably hoping it will come out in the conversation. Or they might wait until the last few minutes and casually toss off, "Oh, by the way. . . ." That's not making the most of the physician's time—or yours.

If you're "turned off" by medical jargon (and it's a legitimate complaint) make sure you know what the doctor is talking about. Ask for explanations in simple language. Don't worry about being a "bother" or asking a "dumb" question. Part of your doctor's job is to put your mind at rest.

Have a specific list of questions in mind before you go in for your appointment. Along with the questions, you should also bring a list of the medicines you may be taking—prescription and over-the-counter preparations. You should be prepared to tell the doctor about any side effects you may have experienced in taking the medicine.

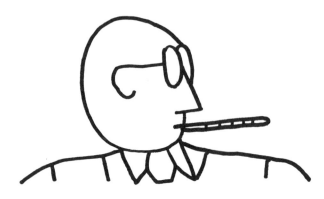

Besides getting right to the point when you are seeing the doctor, be as specific as possible. If possible, don't just say, "I was running a temperature," or "I felt like I was burning up with fever." Keep a thermometer at home and learn how to use it. Then you can report, "Last Tuesday night, my temperature was 100 and two-tenths degrees." Or 99. Or whatever—precisely. (Normal is 98.6 degrees. It's usually indicated by a special mark on the scale to help you find it.)

If you had an ache or pain, try to be specific about where it was located (if it has gone away), when it occurred, what you were doing at the time, how long it lasted, etc.

Some people keep a health notebook. It's a handy way to remember things that happen between visits to the doctor.

When you leave the doctor's office:

- *Know exactly what you are supposed to do, when you are supposed to do it, and why.* As Dr. William B. Stason, associate professor of Health Policy and Management at the Harvard University School of Public Health, wrote recently in the school's *Medical Forum:* "Not only is there no harm in asking why a particular treatment is being given; there can be a good deal of harm in not knowing. For the doctor, this knowledge is often so obvious that it is not mentioned. Talking over a treatment helps the doctor and patient to be sure they're on the same wavelength, and it greatly increases the probability that the treatment will work."

- *Know what to do if you have a question later.* Often a phone call to the doctor's nurse or receptionist can provide you with information if the doctor isn't available. But if you do speak to the doctor, stick to the point. Telephone time generally isn't charged for. Your physician will be grateful for your consideration.

- *Have some definite understanding about a follow-up, whatever the treatment.* Your doctor wants to know if a prescription is working and hasn't caused any problems on its own. Another appointment may not be necessary. Often a phone call or postcard to the office will suffice. Don't stop taking medication too soon because the symptoms have gone away and you feel better, or because of some side effect. The doctor often cares more about some underlying condition than a particular symptom. Ask what to expect from a treatment and for a way to evaluate your progress. Symptoms may be an unreliable clue.

There is no "magic pill" to cure a sour doctor-patient relationship. But trust, confidence, mutual understanding and a willingness to follow your treatment to the letter—all these can help you and your doctor form a good health team.

How to Talk to Your Doctor

How would you like to play a little word game that might help you understand some of those big medical terms your doctor sometimes uses? Let's go.

"Ralphsmithjunior" at first glance is as mind-boggling as "hyperglycemia." But let's separate the two words into their various parts. That's the trick of understanding medical terminology.

In the first word, pick out "smith" in the middle. That's a family name, but there are lots of Smiths. We need to narrow the field, so we add Ralph at the beginning. That's better, but there's a father and son. So, we tack "junior" on the end. Now we know exactly who we're talking about.

Hyperglycemia is a medical term. To understand it, you follow the same process you did when you unraveled "Ralphsmithjunior." In place of Smith, you'll find "glyc" in the middle. That's part of the old Greek word for sweet or sugar. But, just as in the first example, we need to focus more closely. What about the sugar? So, we add "Hyper-" at the beginning. "Hyper-" means above, or beyond, or too much. Now we know that something is too sugary. But what? The ending "-emia" gives us the final clue. It means blood. So that's it. Hyper-glyc-emia means an excess of sugar in the blood. (The opposite of "hyper," incidentally, is "hypo," meaning below or deficient. Hypo-glyc-emia, then, would mean low blood sugar.)

You might ask, "Why don't doctors just say high (or low) blood sugar in the first place?" It's a good question, and there's a good answer. Many of the earliest physicians were Greek, and they were good observers of the human body and its condition. They gave graphic, down-to-earth names to what they saw. Take the old Greek word "karkinos," meaning crab. We still use it today, in a slightly different spelling, for the medical term "carcinoma"—cancer. It would be hard to improve on "crab-like" as a description of a malignant, invading tumor that spreads.

Besides Greek, other medical terms are of Latin origin. The old classical languages are universally understood. They don't have to be translated for the various nationalities. That helps physicians and other health professionals share information around the world. These ancient medical root words are also handy for grafting parts on to help explain the meanings, as we saw in the example of blood sugar.

Here are some other clues to look for as you play medical terminology detective:

"Cardi-" tells you the subject is the heart. Put it together with "electro-" (pertaining to electricity) and "gram-" (from the old Greek word "gramma," meaning writing) and you have electrocardiogram—a graphic record of your heart beat made by an electrical device.

"Enter-" refers to the intestines. Add "-itis" (which means inflamed) and you have "enteritis"—inflammation of the intestines. If the trouble is more extensive, we can add "gastro-" (stomach) and come up with "gastroenteritis"—inflammation of both the stomach and intestines.

"Dys-" at the beginning of a word is not the name of a body part. It tells you that the part that follows isn't working right. It means bad, difficult or painful. Put it in front of "enter," add a "y" on the end, and we have "dysentery"—gut pain that often goes along with inflammation of the intestinal mucous membrane.

Dysmenorrhea is a combination of "dys-" (painful); "men" (month), and "rhea" (flow), with a couple of connecting letters thrown in. So, dysmenorrhea means painful menstruation.

A few other body parts to look for are: "my-" (muscle), "osteo-" (bone), "pneum-" (air) and "pulmo-" (both of which will refer to the lungs).

Here are some endings to remember:

"-ectomy" means that something is going to be removed. Now you know what is meant by "appendectomy" and "tonsillectomy."

"-osis" refers to a diseased condition of the word it is attached to. Used with "scler" to form "sclerosis" we have a hardening condition. Add that combination to "arterio-" (artery) and we have arteriosclerosis—hardening of the arteries.

"-algia" means pain. Neuralgia is nerve pain. Myalgia is muscle pain.

"-oid" on the end of a word means "like." A fibroid tumor is a tumor that looks like fibers. Rheumatoid would mean resembling rheumatism. Rheumatoid arthritis refers to a condition in which inflammation of the joints (like rheumatism) may often be accompanied by marked deformities (as in some arthritis).

A word of caution: Don't try to diagnose an ache or pain just because you know a few medical terms. Use your new understanding, instead, for better communication between you and your doctor. When in doubt, ask questions.

Walking Away from Surgery

Getting out of bed and walking a day or two after surgery, although a fairly standard procedure, still makes some patients uneasy. They probably recall the ordeal a parent, or older friend or relative went through after an operation—the lengthy hospital stay just lying there in bed, sometimes immobilized in a cast. And that, indeed, was the way it was until a medical fluke turned the bed-rest idea topsy-turvy less than 50 years ago.

It happened in Detroit in 1938. A 38-year-old man known to medical history only by the initials R.H. got up and took a walk only hours after an appendectomy, disregarding his doctor's warning about the danger of exercising immediately after surgery.

The next day, the patient felt so well he left the hospital and drove 30 miles to do some errands. He worked in his garden on the third and fourth days after the operation.

Finally, on the fifth day he got in his car again and drove 40 miles to see his surgeon, Dr. Daniel J. Leithauser, for his first medical check-up following the operation.

The surgeon was amazed at R.H.'s speedy convalescence. On the other hand, Leithauser thought, why not? Animals remain active after bearing their young, or undergoing experimental surgery. So he began urging his other appendectomy patients to get out of bed on the first day after an operation. On the second day, provided the patients were willing and felt like it, he discharged them from the hospital. Eventually, the doctor, who was chief surgeon at Detroit's St. Joseph Mercy Hospital, expanded his policy to include all his surgical patients.

The idea didn't catch on fast. Nor was it the first time an American surgeon had advocated early walking exercise after surgery. In 1899, Dr. Emil Ries, a Chicago gynecologist, got most of his patients safely out of bed on the second postoperative day. Still, as Leithauser recalled, the idea was considered by many physicians to be "crackpot." But there are sound arguments for walking soon after surgery, and these have now been accepted.

For one thing, getting out of bed and walking can help to reduce the possibility of blood clots forming in the veins of the legs or pelvis. This can happen during long periods of inactivity. Blood stagnates in the veins of unused leg muscles. If clotting should occur in this sluggish blood, when the patient finally does start to walk a piece of the clot could break away and lodge in the lungs. This could cause a fatal interruption in the circulation.

There's another physiological argument for walking after surgery. A person lying down has a smaller volume of air in the lungs than when standing. There's a simple mechanical reason for this. When you're upright, all the apparatus in your abdominal cavity tends to settle toward the lower end of your trunk. When you lie down, the bowel and other abdominal contents—free somewhat from the downward pull of gravity—tend to push the diaphragm upward.

With less breathing room, the lungs take rapid, shallower breaths. This kind of breathing, particularly in patients who have just had an operation, could lead to two potentially fatal complications—pneumonia and collapse of the air sacs (atelectasis). These risks, while still of grave concern, are more manageable today with antibiotics and respiratory care.

A study of patients who walked immediately after gall bladder surgery showed that one measurement of lung function—called the vital capacity test—returned to normal in less than half the time required by patients who were confined to bed.

Aside from these physiological benefits, getting out of bed and walking soon after surgery does a lot of good for the patient's state of mind. Psychologically, you feel better. And there's an obvious economic gain in being able to get out of the hospital sooner. Leithauser showed that walking cut the length of customary hospitalization in half.

Don't expect to dance a jig. Early walking after surgery, particularly those first few steps, can be painful. But when your doctor suggests trying it, don't think he's being insensitive. He knows what's best for you. Make the effort.

Tips on Taking Medicine

Taking medicine can often become a necessary part of a total program for staying healthy. Some people have to take medicines regularly to control a chronic condition—diabetes, high blood pressure and so on. Others have medicines prescribed for them by a doctor for a temporary bout of illness, or they buy non-prescription medicine at the drug store.

Whatever the case, here are some points to remember about medication, suggested by the Council on Family Health:

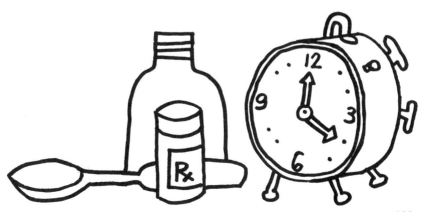

1. If a drug is being prescribed for the first time, or you're buying a medicine you haven't used before, do this:

- Tell your physician, dentist or pharmacist about any other medicines (prescription or non-prescription) you're already taking. Sometimes, when medicines are taken together, the drugs may interact and produce potentially harmful side effects.
- Let them know about any allergies or personal medical conditions you might have, such as diabetes, high blood pressure, pregnancy or glaucoma. Certain personal conditions may mean that it could be harmful to take some drugs, including some you can buy over-the-counter at the drug store.
- Be sure you understand the instructions before leaving the doctor's office or the pharmacy. Does "four times a day" mean "take one every six hours around the clock" or "take four times during your waking hours only"? Should you take the medicine before or after meals? Are there any foods, drinks, activities (such as driving a car or operating machinery) that you should avoid while taking the medicine?

2. When selecting and taking non-prescription medicine, read the label to find out: What symptoms the medicine can relieve; what the active ingredients are; how to take it and how much; when to take it (that's just as important as when *not* to take it); when to stop, and when to consult a doctor. Look for warnings and heed them.

3. When taking prescription medicines, follow the doctor's instructions about how much to take, at what times, and how long to continue.

Sometimes your symptoms will disappear before the conditions that caused them have been totally cleared up. If you stop taking your medicine too soon, your recovery may take longer. Make sure you understand from your doctor how long it's going to take for the medication to do its job. Never take a prescription drug used by a friend or relative. The same medicine may work differently for different people.

4. When taking any medication, prescribed or bought over-the-counter, remember:

- Avoid alcoholic beverages until you check with your doctor or pharmacist. Mixing alcohol and medicines may cause drowsiness, interfere with their effectiveness, or create a potentially dangerous situation.
- Check the expiration date on the medicine label; the medicine may lose its potency or be unsafe to use after the expiration date.
- Throw away all out-of-date medicines; do it safely.
- Keep all medicines in their original containers. This way you'll avoid confusing one medicine with another, and you'll always have the proper instructions at hand.

If a medicine doesn't appear to be working for you, check to make sure you're following all the instructions—how much to take, when to take it, for how long and so on. If the symptoms still hang on, or if there are any new symptoms or unusual side effects, always check with your doctor, dentist, or pharmacist.

Taking medicine, like other parts of a total personal health program—diet, rest, exercise, habits—is your responsibility. When you do your part, you'll probably learn that staying healthy is a lot cheaper and more personally satisfying than simply getting well, desirable as that is when you're sick.

How to Prevent Spreading Viruses

"Dad brought a cold home from work, and now it'll probably run through the whole family."

"There's a lot of that going around."

You've probably heard conversations like that dozens of times. Is it true that an illness can run through a family? Or that large parts of entire communities can be afflicted with some common infectious disease? Very likely.

Infectious diseases—that is, spread from person to person—are caused by germs, either bacterial or viral.

Bacteria are very tiny forms of life. And, just as in real life, there are good guys and bad guys. Many forms of bacteria live usefully and peacefully, causing no harm, in all animals, including humans. They are on our skin, in our noses, mouths, throats and throughout many parts of our bodies. On the other hand, not all bacteria are harmless. There are strains called pathogenic bacteria. These can cause such diseases as diphtheria, whooping cough, scarlet fever, typhoid fever, meningitis and boils.

Viruses are another breed of villain altogether. They are even smaller than bacteria. There are a lot more of them. And once inside the body, they usually cause more trouble. Among the diseases caused by viruses are chicken pox, herpes simplex (including cold sores), measles, mumps, smallpox, mononucleosis, warts, rabies and—yes—the common cold. Viruses are troublesome because they resist most medications.

There are all sorts of ways that people spread both bacteria and viruses among themselves—most commonly perhaps through air and water.

An infected person sheds germs by coughing and sneezing, through body wastes or, in some cases, sexual contact. Other people around pick up the harmful bacteria or viruses in equally diverse ways. They may inhale them. They may ingest them—that is, get them into their systems through the mouth—from contaminated glasses, dishes or food. Or they may come in contact with soiled towels, handkerchiefs, bed linen and so on.

Immunization can prevent many infectious diseases. Children need inoculations against the contagious diseases. Adults can also protect themselves against certain types of influenza germs and some types of pneumonia. Older people, and particularly those with heart and lung ailments, should take special care to protect themselves against infectious diseases.

There are some simple precautions you can take to avoid the kind of comment at the beginning of this column: the cold that has to run its course through the whole family when one member comes down with it:

- Try to avoid contact with any secretion from the sick person's nose, mouth or eyes.
- Try to keep your distance whenever possible. The sick person, preferably, should sleep in a separate room.
- Turn away from coughs and sneezes.
- Don't share food, glasses, utensils or towels.
- Try to use disposable tissues instead of handkerchiefs. Once a tissue has been used, get rid of it.
- Encourage frequent handwashing.

These common sense rules, by themselves, may not keep you from coming down with some of the common afflictions that make the rounds. But they can help.

If you suspect that there's more to it than the sneezing, runny nose and slight fever, check with your doctor. If "there's a lot of it going around," the doctor will know about it and what to do about it.

If You Need a Flu Shot

Should you get a flu shot before winter sets in? The answer depends on your age and general state of health, as well as other considerations best determined between you and your doctor.

Many medical authorities advise flu vaccination for people who fall into several categories. Are you suffering from a chronic illness such as diabetes, heart or kidney disease, anemia? Are you over 65? Are you a heavy smoker? Do you have a breathing problem—asthma, for example? If you answered "yes" to any of those questions, it would probably be a good idea to check with your doctor. Flu vaccination is also considered useful for pregnant women in the second and third trimesters. But, here again, the decision is an individual one between you and your doctor.

There are a couple of important points you should remember about flu vaccines: First, they take about two weeks after injection to become effective. They won't do any good if flu symptoms already have appeared. Second, immunization against known strains of flu virus do not protect you against any new strains which crop up regularly. That's why medical scientists are continually trying to get the jump on this devilish bug that can change its identity from one flu season to the next.

At one time, there probably was a single ancestor of today's family of viruses that cause influenza in humans. And, as in most families, the offspring develop different "personalities," ranging from the relatively inoffensive to the totally malevolent. Influenza C may make you feel generally out of sorts, but is rarely a major health problem. Influenza B can cause large outbreaks and much serious illness, but it is usually far less life-threatening than the really bad apple of the flu virus family. Influenza A is the type that can sweep around the world in a matter of months, causing millions of cases of flu and many thousands of deaths.

Not only is it the worst of the lot, Influenza A is also the most adept quick-change artist, although its kin are also able to switch identities. It is this ability to change that makes one season's flu vaccine relatively ineffective against another winter's flu outbreak. But scientists are beginning to unravel the mystery.

It appears that this variability of the flu virus has something to do with the unusual packaging of the genetic material inside each virus particle. Unlike other viral genetic material, which commonly forms a single continuous strand, the genetic material of flu viruses consist of eight separate pieces of RNA (ribonucleic acid). Each of these pieces contains the codes for one or more of the proteins and other products which the virus needs.

Because the flu's RNA—its identity card—comes in eight pieces, it is believed that this makes it easy for the various pieces to be shuffled around among different flu viruses. But scientists now hope they can make this multi-talented flu virus outsmart itself. One of the main objectives of current research is to find a way to outwit the changeable virus and turn its quick-switch ability into an instrument for its own destruction.

Dr. Edwin D. Kilbourne of Mt. Sinai School of Medicine in New York, an internationally known expert on influenza, believes this is possible.

He thinks the flu's variability someday might be used to develop strains that would be highly infectious, but whose infections would be harmless. This is the case now with some live-virus vaccines against other diseases. Such viruses, Kilbourne believes, might replace or even change the dangerous "wild" viruses that have always afflicted mankind.

No discussion of cold weather health hazards would be complete without mention of the common cold although the cold weather, by itself, doesn't *cause* colds. Colds also are caused by a virus—any one of more than 100 different strains, many of which we harbor at all times. We "catch cold" more often in the winter most likely because we're in closer contact with other people, usually indoors. And colds are spread by people who already have colds—by coughing or sneezing or in close conversation.

Once you have a cold, there's little to do about it except to rest as much as possible, make yourself comfortable, and let the body's natural defense against infection do its job. Generally, this takes a week or two. Meanwhile, expectorants and nasal decongestants may help to ease breathing difficulties. Aspirin is effective in relieving headaches and malaise, that pooped-out feeling.

A Home Emergency Center

Most home medicine cabinets are a mess, a ridiculous hodgepodge of assorted beauty aids, old razor blades, shaving cream, nail polish, hair pins, unused vitamins, outdated prescriptions—you name it. This is as absurd as it is untidy. It makes no sense because an estimated one out of three visits to hospital emergency rooms could be avoided if people had a well-stocked medicine cabinet and a basic working knowledge of how and when to use the contents.

Sylvia Porter, the financial columnist, says that for an investment of as little as $35 you can stock your medicine cabinet to prepare yourself to handle the most common minor illnesses and household accidents. And Dr. George Royer of the Upjohn Co., the Michigan-based pharmaceuticals maker, calls the medicine cabinet "the home's medical emergency treatment center for illnesses and injuries that happen when you least expect them."

Why not take on this job as part of your spring housecleaning? It will be time and money well spent. First, clean out all those items that have outlived their usefulness. Check the expiration dates on all medicines, prescription and non-prescription. If there are any that are out-of-date,

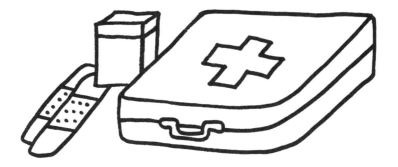

toss them out. Keep only the medicines you are using now for chronic conditions, such as high blood pressure, arthritis or asthma.

Now you're ready to sensibly re-stock your cleared-out cabinet. Here are some typical home emergencies, and suggestions for supplies to help you cope with them:

Minor cuts and scrapes. Get an antiseptic for cleaning the wound, and an antibiotic to apply afterward. Ask your druggist what he would recommend. You'll also need sterile gauze or bandages to keep out dirt and germs.

Eye injuries. Plain tap water may be your best bet for flushing out foreign particles that get in the eye. If that doesn't work, make a patch out of the sterile gauze and get medical attention.

Minor skin irritations. A hydrocortisone skin preparation can temporarily relieve the itch and redness that go along with dermatitis, eczema, or "dishpan hands." You won't need a prescription. Ask your druggist for suggestions. These skin preparations, incidentally, also are helpful for such summertime aggravations as mild poison ivy and insect bites.

Minor burns. Cold tap water is your best first step. Follow that with a burn ointment—possibly. However, if the burn is deep, don't use an ointment. The doctor will just have to scrape it off later before he can treat the burn. And no matter what you've heard about home-remedy old wives' tales—never put butter on a burn.

Swallowed poisons. In some cases, syrup of ipecac can be used to induce vomiting after an overdose of drugs or medication. However, don't use it if the swallowed substance is an acid-based poison or strong alkali such as drain cleaner. Call your local poison control center immediately. Have the label on the container handy so you can tell the poison control center what was swallowed. Follow instructions.

There are some other essential items you should have on hand: Aspirin, antacid tablets, elastic bandages for sprains, cough syrup, tongue depressors, petroleum jelly, blunt-end scissors, thermometer, sterile cotton balls and gauze pads.

Finally, write down important health service phone numbers: hospital, poison control center, physician, emergency squad. Put one copy of the list near the medicine cabinet, and another near the telephone.

These measures won't keep you from getting sick or having an accident around the house. But they can take care of many minor emergencies, maybe save you a trip to the hospital, or put you in better shape for going—if that's necesary.

Planning for Retirement

One of the health hazards the great majority of all workers eventually must face, regardless of age or occupation, is retirement. Like other hazards of the workplace, you can either learn how to cope with it and not get hurt, or you can bang into it unprepared and suffer.

Joe wasn't prepared. One day he realized with a shock that he was just about a year away from retirement age. He began to worry about his approaching loss of status from the oldest and most respected worker on the shift—the guy the young fellows looked up to—to just another idle old man. His productivity dropped. He began to mess up more material. There were more days lost because of sickness or accident. Joe became quarrelsome with his fellow workers and his supervisors. He was about to barge into retirement unprepared and he was suffering—physically and emotionally.

Marge prepared. About 10 years ago, in her late 40s, she started having regular medical checkups. She also made a list of things she might be able to learn how to do after that inevitable day—retirement. Later, she sought counseling provided by her union. She became involved in community activities. Marge had a plan. The "hazard" was still there. But she was learning how to cope when it arose and make the transition reasonably unscathed.

Retirement can affect two aspects of your total health: your physical health, and your mental health. Ideally, a worker should begin to plan for his or her retirement at least five or 10 years beforehand. It might well begin with an evaluation of health status.

Some of the first symptoms of chronic disabling illness begin to show up between the ages of 40 and 50. Chronic diseases—cancer and those of the heart, kidney, and blood vessels—account for most of the illnesses of older people, although there are no particular diseases limited to old age. The elderly also are more likely to come down with pneumonia, influenza and other respiratory infections.

By paying careful attention to physical health during your earlier

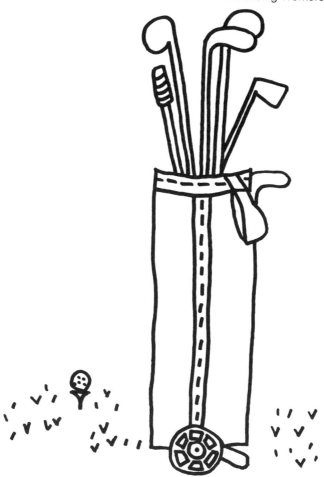

years, these chronic diseases lying in wait down the road a few years hence might be more completely under control for a more enjoyable retirement.

An important part of keeping well, particularly among older people, is nutrition. Older people tend toward malnutrition for a number of possible reasons: ignorance; lack of funds to buy wholesome foods; long-established poor eating habits; poor appetite, often caused by low morale; and because a lot of older people cook and eat alone.

Learning about nutrition can be a double blessing for those planning for retirement. It can help them maintain good health and a sense of well-being, as well as provide another interest to help replace a job-related interest. You can replace a no longer used skill to maintain a machine by learning how to care for a much more complicated machine—your body.

191

Mental health can be affected by retirement because all of us need to be needed. Too many retirees think of themselves as no longer needed. These people suffer a great deal of mental and emotional stress. They can help themselves by broadening their interests while they are still working and drawing up a plan.

If there is a magic key to well-being in your later years, it would be "keeping active." Work itself is a powerful medicine. If you don't have to retire, and if your health permits, keep working—perhaps at a reduced pace and with fewer responsibilities.

If retirement is mandatory and you have to leave your job, here are some tips on how to keep active:

- Be specific, not just "fishing" or "travel."
- Choose something you would like to do, and *must* do, on a regular schedule, not just when you feel like it.
- Set reasonable goals—part time, even volunteer work. While certainly a consideration for many people, earnings at this point are not the main thing. More important is the regular performance of a job that is useful to somebody else as well as yourself.
- If there doesn't seem to be anything else but your job that interests you, ask for help through pre-retirement counseling.

Too many ill-prepared retirees slip into a decline because they stop trying new activities. When they do that, they stop growing. Growth is a result of assuming responsibilities and obligations. Retirement, all too often, is the start of decay and untimely death.

But it doesn't have to be that way. Start planning for retirement early. And make your plan cover all phases of life—physical, mental, social, economic, work, play, and worship. It can be rewarding.

HMOs—One Way to Control Costs

The cost of keeping Americans healthy is rising steadily year after year. What can be done to contain this cost?

Because employee health care has become a big cost of doing business, it is coming under closer scrutiny by managements looking for ways to control their rising expenditures. An employer, for instance, may seek to cut his health insurance premiums by going for a package with larger deductibles. But that kind of savings comes at the worker's expense. You have to shell out more out-of-pocket money before your benefits begin.

Understandably, labor looks upon this as a "takeaway" of gains it has been able to negotiate for union members. So the options of higher deductibles or reduced benefits are not very pleasant as ways to curb rising health care costs. At best they are unpopular. At worst, they can embitter the bargaining process.

Is there a better way? The answer is a qualified "probably yes." The alternative many businesses and industries—both large and small—are looking into is something called Health Maintenance Organizations, HMOs for short.

The main idea of HMOs is early diagnosis and preventive treatment. Experience has shown that this approach can reduce the need, in many cases, for hospitalization. And this alone can take a big chunk out of the nation's annual health care bill.

However, HMOs are not a stripped-down benefit package. The coverage is comprehensive, including both hospitalization and out-patient services. Care is available 24 hours a day, seven days a week. The services are provided on a fixed monthly prepaid fee. Some companies have set up their own in-house HMOs. Others have chosen to go another way, forming a corporate relationship with an existing HMO that serves the community at large.

Congress passed the HMO Act in 1973 as a means of seeing whether health care costs might be reduced. The law applies to workers who already are covered by some form of group health insurance or other health benefits package. When an HMO presents a valid request to be included in such a company's health care plans, the employer must give the workers an option: Stay put, or join the HMO and pay an amount equal to whatever is paid under the company plan.

Actually, there is a triple option: The company plan, the HMO or an IPA—or Individual Practice Association which is also recognized under the law. The law also provides funding for planning and start-up costs for IPAs and HMOs.

The HMOs and the IPAs differ in some important ways. In general, the HMO or "closed panel" involves physicians practicing together under one roof who are either part of a medical "group," pooling their income, or who are on salary and part of the HMO staff. The IPA, on the other hand, is an "open panel" in which the physicians practice in their own offices, not a centralized facility, and are part of an organized system of health care with coordination of referral and hospital care. Both types of organizations have demonstrated that they can cut health care costs by reducing the number of hospital stays per 1,000 members to about half the national average.

IPAs tend to be popular with both physicians and workers. For the doctors, the system involves little change from their regular practice. For

193

the patients, it may be easier to go to the doctor's office instead of a centralized location. There is also the likelihood of maintaining an already established doctor-patient relationship.

The cost effectiveness of HMOs depends to a large extent on the unit's control of facilities it operates. A basic problem for the IPAs is also one of control over the expensive elements of the system—the facilities, overhead, equipment and the like.

One major problem of HMOs is in fitting the operation into a company with employers who may be scattered over the country in regional plants and offices. One idea that has been studied is a network of coordinated HMOs to which dispersed employees could turn while they are away from the parent company. There are other knotty issues such as rates which may vary in different locations, the different levels of benefits between different HMOs, transfer of memberships and so on.

But the fact that HMOs are in existence, that for almost a decade they have been demonstrating an ability to hold down the high cost of health care and, most important, that employers are finally taking a careful look at an idea that offers the possibility of savings without cutting benefits—all of these are encouraging developments.

HMOs may not yet be the whole answer to a very complex problem. But they are showing that enlightened cooperation can have a manifold beneficial effect: in compassionate care at a bearable cost and by providing choices that offer more harmony in union-management relationships.

A Local Union Tackles Health Costs

What can unions do to help control ever-mounting health care costs? Some possibile answers may be suggested by a recent survey of medical claims to the Health and Welfare Trust Fund of a local union in California. The International Union of Operating Engineers (IUOE), Local 3, in the San Francisco Bay area wanted to find out, among other things, if there existed any possible relationship between jobs and health claims, and whether workers who were found to have a potential disease problem in a screening program sought follow-up medical care.

Here are some of the findings in that survey:

- Operators of heavy equipment have an apparent higher potential risk of developing liver and kidney problems.
- Heavy equipment operators have a noise-induced hearing loss, a

conclusion borne out by the fact that the loss is greater in the left ear (nearest the open window of the cab).

- Only about one-third of the persons who took part in the union-based screening made a health claim related to a positive finding within a year after the screening.

The first two of these findings suggest an immediate need to install "environmental cabs" in heavy equipment to protect operators from the effects of both vibration and noise. The last finding suggests that the benefits of health screening—both in reducing illnesses and costs—will be realized only if workers seek health care for a potential condition that has been brought to their attention. Otherwise, the whole purpose of health screening is defeated.

This survey of IUOE Local 3's medical claims was conducted by the Western Institute for Occupational/Environmental Sciences (WIOES), Berkeley, Calif. As a result of the study, WIOES recommended that Local 3 develop a union-based health maintenance program to improve the health of its members and cut costs—for members, the trust fund, and employers alike.

While unions differ greatly as to the industries, trades and occupations they cover, some of the key elements in the proposal to Local 3, IUOE, might well be adaptable to others. These elements include:

- Compilation of baseline data from which any relationships between jobs and diseases can be studied, based on health claims.
- Computer entry of data in such a manner that periodic and on-going analyses can be made.
- A health promotion program, including assistance to members in: smoking cessation, weight control, diet and nutrition, substance abuse, accident prevention in the home, medical self-care, wiser buying and using of medical care, prescription drugs and elective surgery; prenatal and child care; marital and family counseling.
- A computer-based "early warning system" to detect health effects or health changes in a given group, with provisions for follow-ups so that medical intervention may slow or stop the progress of disease.

WIOES also recommended that Local 3 adopt a plan for a health maintenance program using two groups for comparison purposes over a five-year period to see if such a program can keep members healthier and trim costs.

The thinking behind health maintenance programs is both humanistic and economic. Workers and their families can enjoy the advantages of increased longevity, higher family income and financial stability, and

195

general improvement in the quality of life associated with good health. A well-designed health maintenance and promotion program appears to be an excellent service for a union to provide for its members.

Health Care in 21st Century America

What will health care be like 20, 30, 50 years into the future? Based on continued progress in medical research and technology, here are some of the things you might be reading about in the 21st century.

The so-called "hospital-on-the-wrist" is available in stores. This is a tiny medical computer that can monitor body functions and—when necessary—begin appropriate drug or electromagnetic treatment.

Artificial blood is used widely for emergency transfusions. The emulsion, developed from earlier experiments with fluorocarbons, performs all the main functions of hemoglobin. It is routinely used in open-heart procedures, and by ambulance personnel transporting accident victims.

Burn treatment has been revolutionized by the development of a synthetic membrane that breathes like human skin, yet is so fine it prevents liquids and bacteria from passing through.

Medical specialists can now cause bone and tissue to grow back—regenerate themselves—by using electromagnetic stimulation. If the damage is beyond repair, there is a nationwide chain of spare-parts banks for humans.

Organ transplants, gene therapy and telemedicine are commonplace in the 21st century. An anti-aging vaccine is widely used. The breakthrough came with recognition that senile dementia was caused by a virus.

"Smart" pills have been developed. These are microscopic globules of latex coated with antibodies. They're called "smart" because they can be instructed to seek out and attack antigens of a specific tumor cell. Highly discriminating, the tiny vehicles are useful in targeting cancer or other unwanted cells with lethal drugs or radioactive elements without endangering nearby healthy tissue.

Screening for genetic markers—by the year 2032 a standard procedure for the entire population—can identify in infancy what diseases a child will be susceptible to in later life. Armed with this information, an individual can chart his or her optimal lifestyle and occupational choices.

Fifty years from now, you'll probably see many changes in industry and the workplace:

- Occupational hazard control plans for all new processes, equipment and installations are subject to pre-evaluation and approval under a national regulatory program.
- Comprehensive health care delivery systems, including occupational health programs for employees and their families, have been established through legislative and private sector labor-management initiatives.
- A national computerized early warning system for instantly monitoring adverse pharmacological chemical effects is operational.
- More accurate and reliable screening tests—enzymatic, immunological, electronic, etc.—can diagnose a wide range of hazards. These tests can point the finger at substances that can cause cancer, damage to the nervous system, alter our genes or cause birth defects. In the 21st century, such tests have become part of an ongoing and routine medical monitoring system.
- Health education curricula include concepts of occupational illness and injury, including the roles of lifestyles, personal habits and individual hazard exposure levels.

As health care monitoring and information networks spread, the era of the small industrial clinic is coming to an end.

There are some somber tones in this otherwise bright picture. If some futurists are correct, technological progress can carry a price tag. The 21st century could see an increase in stress-related illnesses. Mental illness and drug and alcohol abuse may persist as serious problems.

There is also, of course, one critical factor not mentioned in these projections: the national economy. If the economic cycles continue to leave us with ever-higher levels of unemployment, denying productive work to many millions of people, then all bets on the future could be off.

But, on balance, the future of health care is hopeful and exciting, if the present pace can be sustained. The greatest advance may not be some marvelous tool or spectacular procedure. Instead, it may well be a growing awareness by people that they have the right to a safe and healthful workplace, that it is achievable and they can help make it so.

Glossary

A

ANTIBIOTIC A substance produced by living organisms such as bacteria, or molds, which can destroy other bacteria. Penicillin is the most familiar example. Some antibiotics have shown effective anticancer activity.

ANTIBODY A substance formed by the body as a reaction to a foreign agent or antigen. The antibody formed works only against that particular antigen.

ANTIGEN Any foreign substance which causes the formation of antibodies as protective substances in the body.

ASBESTOS A mineral that appears in a fibrous and fluffy form when separated from rock in the asbestos mining process.

ASBESTOS-RELATED DISEASES All those states of ill health that arise out of, or are associated with, past exposure to asbestos. These include:

Asbestosis An incurable scarring of the lungs caused by asbestos fibers lodging in the lungs. The fibers irritate the lung causing inflammation. As the inflammation heals, it leaves scar tissue that potentially impedes at a gradual rate the flow of oxygen from the lungs into the bloodstream. The result can be slow suffocation or heart failure. Asbestosis may develop within 15-20 years with moderate exposures.

Lung cancer Lung cancer usually takes 20-30 years to develop in asbestos workers and exposure must be over a long period of time.

Mesothelioma A rare cancer of the membrane lining the lungs or abdominal cavity which is associated mainly with exposure to asbestos. Even mini-mal exposure (two months) can cause the disease 20-30 years later.

Cancers elsewhere in the body usually appear 20-40 years after exposure. Cancers may affect the stomach, large intestine, kidney, larynx, or rectum.

ASPHYXIANTS Volatile substances which induce anoxemia or an equivalent condition. They interfere with either the supply or the utilization of oxygen.

AT RISK An individual or group, who because of particular biological, lifestyle and/or occupational/environmental exposures, have an increased likelihood of developing a disease or disability. This individual or population is said to be at risk for that disability/disease due to the presence of any one or combination of the above-mentioned factors. See also "Risk Factors."

B

BARIUM ENEMA The use of barium sulfate introduced into the intestinal tract by an enema to allow X-ray exam of the lower bowel.

BASAL CELL CARCINOMA The most common type of skin cancer. It forms in the lowermost layer of the skin, grows slowly and seldom spreads. It is easily detected and readily cured when treated promptly.

BENIGN TUMOR An abnormal swelling or growth that is not a cancer and is usually harmless.

BIOCHEMISTRY The study of the chemical structure and the chemical function of all living organisms.

BIOPSY The surgical removal of a piece of tissue from a living subject for microscopic examination to make a diagnosis, e.g., to determine whether cancer cells are present.

BLOOD COUNT An examination of the blood to count the number of white and red blood cells and platelets.

BREAST SELF-EXAMINATION Simple procedure to examine breasts thoroughly, recommended once a month for all women to do themselves between regular physician checkups.

BYSSINOSIS One of the dust diseases; it is often called the brown lung disease. Whatever the name, cotton dust, flax or hemp, breathed into the lungs over a period of time, may harm the lungs.

C

CANCER A large group of diseases characterized by uncontrolled growth and spread of abnormal cells.

CARCINOGEN Any substance that causes cancer.

Known carcinogens Those carcinogens that have been demonstrated to definitely produce cancer in humans.

Suspect carcinogens Compounds implicated in human cancer or shown to be carcinogenic in lab animals.

CARCINOMA A form of cancer which arises in the tissues that cover or line such organs of the body as skin, intestines, uterus, lung, breast, etc.

CARCINOMA IN SITU A stage in the growth of cancer when it is still confined to the tissue in which it started.

CELL The basic structural unit of life.

CERVIX Any neck or neck-like structure in the body; in cancer terminology it usually refers to the neck of the uterus.

CHEMOTHERAPY Treatment of disease by chemical compounds.

CHRONIC CONDITION A condition which is long and drawn out in duration and usually incurable.

CLINICAL Pertaining to the study and treatment of disease in human beings by direct observation, as distinguished from laboratory research.

CO-CARCINOGEN When carcinogens are present together and enhance the action of each other.

COLON The part of the large intestine that extends from the end of the small intestine to the rectum.

COLONOSCOPY Technique for direct visual examination of the entire large bowel by means of a lighted, flexible tube.

COLOSTOMY A surgical procedure which creates an artificial opening from the colon through the abdominal wall in order to permit elimination of wastes.

COLPOSCOPY Examination of the vagina and cervix with a magnifying instrument called a colposcope to check prestained tissues for abnormality.

COMBINATION THERAPY The use of two or more modes of treatment—surgery, irradiation, chemotherapy, immunotherapy — in combination, alternately or together, to achieve optimum results against cancer.

CYTOLOGY The science which deals with the study of living cells. Cells which have been sloughed off, or scraped off, from such organs of the body as uterus, lungs, bladder or stomach are examined under the microscope for early signs of abnormality. The Pap test used for early detection of cervical cancer is an example of this method; also referred to as exfoliative cytology.

CYST   An abnormal sac which contains a liquid or semisolid material; may be benign or malignant.

D

DIAGNOSIS   Identifying a disease by its signs, symptoms, course and laboratory findings.

DUSTS   A collection of small, dry organic or inorganic particles formed when solid matter is broken down by natural and mechanical forces and are fine enough to remain suspended in the air for some time if disturbed.

DOSE-RESPONSE   Reactive site produces response which is related to concentration at active site. Concentration at active site is related to dose.

E

ENDOMETRIAL   Having to do with the lining of the uterus or body of the womb, used in describing a form of uterine cancer.

ENTEROSTOMAL THERAPIST   An allied health professional trained in the care of stomas, or openings in the abdominal wall, constructed to permit the elimination of wastes from the digestive or urinary tracts.

ENVIRONMENTAL CANCER   Cancer caused, in part, by carcinogens present in the general surroundings or encountered in enclosed settings such as in the home, school or workplace. See also "Occupational Cancer."

EMPHYSEMA   A lung disease, in which the walls of the air sacs (alveoli) have been stretched too thin and broken down.

ENVIRONMENT-HOST-AGENT   A basic model of public health science. This model, called the Epidemiologic Triangle, states that an ecological approach is necessary to explain the occurrence of disease; disease cannot be attributed to the operation of any one factor.

ENZYME   A complex organic compound produced in the body capable of speeding up a particular chemical reaction.

EPIDEMIOLOGY   The study of incidence, distribution, environmental causes and control of a disease in a population.

ESOPHAGEAL SPEECH   An acquired technique by which laryngectomees (those who have lost their voice boxes) are taught to speak again by swallowing and expelling air through the mouth from the esophagus (gullet).

ESTROGEN   A hormone secreted by the ovaries which is essential to reproduction; involved in the menstrual cycle; produces female secondary sex characteristics, such as breast development.

ETIOLOGY   The study of the causes of disease.

EXCISION   Surgical removal of a diseased part of the body, including cancerous growths.

EXCORIATION   Break in skin surface, usually covered with blood or serous crusts.

F

FUMES   Suspension of very fine (less than 1.0 micron) solid particles in air. The term usually applies to freshly-formed oxides of metals, such as zinc, iron and magnesium.

G

GASES   Fluids which normally occupy the space of enclosure and which can be changed to the liquid or solid state only by the combined effect of increased pressure and decreased temperature. Also: A compound which is in the gaseous state under normal conditions.

GENES   The hereditary units of life which control the cell's transfer of a trait or process.

GUAIAC TEST   A chemical test used to detect occult (hidden) blood in the stool. A simple method allows stool specimens to be placed on special guaiac-treated paper slides. These slides are then treated and checked by a doctor or lab technician. The test is well-suited to screening programs for colon-rectal cancer because the specimen can be prepared at home.

GOVERNMENT B READER   A physician who has had specialized training in the interpretation of chest X rays for dusty lung disease and who passed a test given by the American College of Physicians/NIOSH.

H

HAZARDS   Likelihood that substance will cause injury under conditions of use.

HEALTH   A state of complete physical, mental and social well-being and not merely the absence of disease or infirmity.

HODGKIN'S DISEASE   A form of cancer that affects the lymphatic system—the network of glands or nodes and vessels which manufactures and circulates lymph throughout the body to fight infection.

HORMONES   Chemicals that help regulate the body mechanisms including growth, metabolism and reproduction.

HORMONOTHERAPY   Treatment by the use of hormones; used in controlling cancers in conjunction with other modalities such as chemotherapy.

HYSTERECTOMY   A surgical procedure for removal of the uterus; may be combined with removal of ovaries (oophorectomy).

I

ILEOSTOMY   A surgical procedure which constructs an artificial opening of the small intestine through the abdominal wall for elimination of body wastes.

IMMUNOLOGY   Branch of science dealing with the body's resistance mechanism against disease or the invasion of a foreign substance.

IMMUNOTHERAPY   Treatment of disease by stimulating the body's own defense mechanism against the disease.

INDUSTRIAL HYGIENIST   The professional concerned with preventive medicine at the worksite. The industrial hygienist's functions are: recognition, evaluation and control of health hazards in the work environment and training and education of employers and employees.

IRRITANTS   Gases which would be regarded as corrosives. They injure the tissues of the respiratory tract, and they induce inflammation of the air passages or the lungs.

L

LARYNGECTOMY   A surgical procedure which removes the larynx or voice box. A laryngectomee is someone who has undergone this surgery.

LATENCY PERIOD   The time which elapses between exposure to a carcinogen and the first manifestation of damage.

LESION   Describes any abnormal change in tissue due to disease or injury.

LEUKEMIA   Cancer of the blood-forming tissues (bone marrow, lymph nodes, spleen); characterized by the overproduction of white blood cells.

LUNG CANGER   A malignant growth in the lung tissue.

LYMPH A clear fluid which circulates throughout the body, containing white blood cells called lymphocytes, antibodies and nourishing substances.

LYMPH GLAND Tissue which is made up of lymphocytes and connective tissue and produces lymph and lymphocytes (also called lymph node). These lymph glands, or nodes, normally act as filters for impurities in the body.

LYMPHEDEMA Swelling as a result of obstruction of lymphatic vessels or lymph nodes.

LYMPHOMA Malignant growths of lymph nodes.

M

MALIGNANT Leading toward progressive invasion of body tissues and probably ending in death. Generally, the tumor invades nearby tissues and spreads to other parts of the body.

MALIGNANT TUMOR A tumor made up of cancer cells. These tumors continue to grow and invade surrounding tissues; cells may break away and grow elsewhere. (See Benign Tumor, Metastasis)

MAMMOGRAPHY Low-dose X-ray technique for studying the structure of breast tissue in order to locate any abnormality at the earliest possible stage; permits detection of a breast cancer before the lump can be felt.

MASTECTOMY Surgical removal of a cancerous breast to prevent spread of the disease. Simple mastectomy refers to removal of the entire breast. Radical mastectomy involves removal of the entire breast, underlying muscle tissue and lymph nodes in the armpit. A mastectomee is someone who has had the breast removed.

MELANOMA A pigmented, highly malignant form of cancer of the skin. The tumor may vary in color from nearly black to almost white.

MESOTHELIOMA A rare cancer of the membrane lining of the lungs or abdominal cavity which is associated mainly with exposure to asbestos.

METASTASIS The process by which cancer cells break away and spread to other places in the body by way of the lymph and blood systems and start new malignant tumors.

MISTS Suspended liquid droplets generated by condensation from the gaseous to the liquid state or by breaking up a liquid into a dispersed state, such as by splashing, foaming, and atomizing.

MICROMETER 1/25,000 of an inch or 1,000 of a millimeter.

MITOSIS The process of cell reproduction by which new cells are formed.

MUTAGEN Anything that causes a mutation. Most carcinogens are also mutagens. Testing a substance to see if it is a mutagen may turn out to be a fairly reliable way to see if it is a carcinogen. Such tests are easier, faster, and cheaper than the usual animal tests since they can be done with bacteria.

MUTATION A change in genetic make-up that can be passed from generation to generation.

N

NEOPLASM Any new abnormal growth of cells or issues; may be benign or malignant but is customarily used to describe a cancerous tumor.

O

OCCUPATIONAL CANCER Cancer caused by carcinogens present in the work environment or encountered during performance of the job.

OCCUPATIONAL HEALTH HISTORY A comprehensive chronology of an individual's place of employment, toxic exposures and work environments.

OCCUPATIONAL PHYSICIAN A physician who has advanced training in the diagnosis, treatment and prevention of diseases arising out of the workplace.

ONCOLOGY The study of cancer, which has become a specialty branch of modern medicine.

OSTOMY A surgical procedure that creates a stoma, or artificial opening. A stoma of the intestinal and urinary tracts permits the elimination of wastes through the abdominal wall. A stoma of the respiratory tract permits the passage of air through the neck. An ostomate is someone who has had this form of surgery.

P

PALLIATIVE TREATMENT Providing relief from symptoms of a disease but not directly curing the disease; alleviating pain.

PALPATION A detection procedure using the hands to examine organs without the aid of instruments.

PAP TEST Developed by the late Dr. George Papanicolaou, to examine, under the microscope, cells found in vaginal secretions. Its major purpose is to detect cancer of the cervix in its earliest stage. (See Cytology)

PATHOLOGY The science which studies the nature, cause and development of disease through examination of tissues and fluids of the body. A pathologist does autopsies and examines urine, blood, tissues removed for biopsies, etc.

PELVIC EXAMINATION Examination of the organs of the pelvis, through the vagina and rectum.

PLATELETS A small circular or oval disk present in blood which is necessary for the ability of the blood to clot and/or retract.

PNEUMOCONIOSIS 1. A fibrous hardening of the lungs caused by the irritation created from the inhalation of dust. The kind of dust inhaled determines the type of condition or injury. Also 2. A class of dusty lung diseases, of which the following are included in this category of pneumoconioses (as examples): asbestosis, byssinosis, silicosis. (See also Asbestosis, Byssinosis, Silicosis)

PNEUMONECTOMY A surgical procedure for removal of an entire lung.

POISON Any substance that causes injury, illness, or death, especially by chemical means.

POLYP An overgrowth of tissue projecting into a cavity of the body, e.g., the lining of the colon, the nasal passage, or the surface of vocal cords.

PREVENTIVE MEDICINE Seeks to prevent a person from becoming ill. General methods for accomplishing this are education, eliminating hazards, establishing improved work practices for preventive reasons, and requiring regular physical examinations.

PROCTO Short for proctosigmoidoscopy, an examination of the first 10 inches of the rectum and colon with a hollow, lighted tube.

PROGNOSIS Prediction of the course of a disease and the future prospects for the patient.

PROSTATE A gland located at the base of the bladder in males.

PROSTHESIS An artificial replacement for a missing body part, e.g., breast form, leg, arm, eye.

PROTOCOL Standardized procedures followed by physicians so that results of treatment of different patients can be compared.

PULMONARY SPECIALIST A physician with formalized training in the diagnosis and treatment of lung disorders.

R

RADIATION THERAPY Treatment of cancer with radiant energy of extremely short wavelengths which damages or kills cancer cells. Radioactive elements such as cobalt 60, radium and radon, gallium and cesium 27 are used to produce gamma rays. Supervoltage machines, such as betatrons and linear accelerators are used as sources of X rays.

RADIOLOGIST A physician with special experience using radiant energy in the diagnosis and treatment of disease.

REGIONAL INVOLVEMENT When cancer has spread from its original site to nearby areas. (See Metastasis)

REMISSION Complete or partial disappearance of the signs and symptoms of a disease; or the period during which a disease is under control.

RISK FACTORS Factors whose presence is associated with an increased likelihood that disease will develop at a later time. (Example: smoking and heavy asbestos exposure are risk factors which, when combined, increase an individual's risk of developing asbestosis or lung cancer 92 times.)

S

SARCOMA A form of cancer that arises in the connective tissue and muscles, such as bone and cartilage.

SILICOSIS A disease of the lungs caused by the inhalation of finely divided free silica dust. Where silica dust accumulates, a fibrous tissue develops and grows around the particle. It is not as elastic as normal lung tissue, and does not permit the ready passage of oxygen and carbon dioxide.

SMOKE Carbon or soot particles less than 0.1 micron in size which result from the incomplete combustion of carbonaceous materials such as coal, oil, tar, and tobacco.

SPUTUM TEST A study of cells from the lungs contained in material coughed up in the sputum.

STAGING Determining the extent of growth of a cancer so that results of treatment can be compared and prognosis offered.

STRESS A physical, chemical or emotional factor that causes bodily or mental tension and may be a factor in disease causation or fatigue.

SYNERGISM Cooperative action of substances whose total effect is greater than the sum of their separate effects.

T

TERATOGEN An agent which, when administered to a pregnant female, results in damage to the developing offspring.

THERAPY The treatment of disease.

THERMOGRAPHY A technique for measuring the surface temperature of parts of the body to detect underlying disease; used along with mammography and palpation for discovering breast cancer in its earliest stage.

TISSUE A collection of similar cells. There are four basic tissues in the body: 1) epithelial, 2) connective, 3) muscle, 4) nerve.

THRESHOLD LIMIT VALUE (TLV) An exposure level under which most people can work consistently for eight hours a day, day after day, with no harmful effects.

TOXICITY A relative property of a chemical agent and refers to a harmful effect on some biologic mechanism and the condition under which this effect occurs.

TOXICOLOGY The study of the nature, effects and detection of poisons and the treatment of poisoning.

TRACHEOSTOMY A surgical procedure to create a stoma or permanent opening of the trachea or windpipe through the neck. Tracheotomy is the surgery that temporarily provides direct passage of air into the windpipe.

TUMOR A swelling or enlargement; an abnormal mass, either benign or malignant, which performs no useful body function.

V

VAPORS 1. The gaseous form of substances normally in the solid or liquid state, which can be changed to these states either by increasing the pressure or decreasing the temperature alone. Also 2. A compound which is normally a solid or liquid but becomes gaseous under other conditions.

VIROLOGY The branch of biology dealing with the study of viruses.

VIRUS A tiny living parasite which invades cells and alters their chemistry so that the cells are compelled to produce more virus particles. Viruses cause many diseases.

W

WORK DISABILITY A health or physical condition, arising out of the workplace, which hinders a person in work activity. Such a disability may be partial or complete.

WORKER'S COMPENSATION Federal and state programs designed to provide cash benefits and medical care to workers injured or diseased in connection with their work, and payments to the survivors of those who sustain fatal injuries or diseases.

WORKER'S COMPENSATION ATTORNEYS

Applicants' attorney A lawyer who specializes in the processing of a claim on behalf of an injured/diseased worker. These claims are generally processed through the worker's compensation or criminal system.

Defense attorney A lawyer either employed or retained by a company to defend against a legal suit brought forth by an injured/diseased worker.

X

XERORADIOGRAPHY A photographic way of recording X-ray images; useful in detecting breast cancer early.

X RAY Radiant energy of extremely short wavelength, used to diagnose and treat cancer.

Scientific Terms

cc   cubic centimeter (equal to 0.06 of a cubic inch

g   gram (equal to 1/1000 of a kilogram)

kg   kilogram (equal to approximately 2.2 pounds)

mg   milligram (equal to 1/1000 gram)

μg   microgram (equal to 1/1000 milligram)

mg/m³   microgram per cubic meter

ppb   parts per billion (1 ppb = one ten-millionth of one percent)

ppm   parts per million (1 ppm = one ten-thousandth of one percent)

ppt   parts per trillion (1 ppt = one thousandth of a ppb)

rad   the present standard unit of radioactive dose

rem   meaning Roentgen Equivalent Man; the amount of ionizing radiation required to produce the same biological effect as one roentgen of high penetration X rays

Roentgen   a unit of radioactive dose or exposure; that amount of X or gamma radiation that will produce an electrostatic unit of charge in one cubic centimeter of dry air at standard temperature and pressure

millirem   one one-thousandth of a roentgen (rem). In general, for population groups, the federal recommended limit is 170 millirems per year to the average individual. This limit is about twice the natural background radiation to which everyone is unavoidably exposed: an average of 84 millirems per person annually in the United States.

α particle   also known as alpha ray, alpha radiation; a small electrically charged particle of very high velocity thrown off by many radioactive materials, including uranium and radium. It is made up of two neutrons and two protons. Its electric charge is positive and twice as great as that of an electron.

β particle   also known as beta radiation; a small electrically charged particle thrown off by many radioactive materials. It is identical with the electron and possesses the smallest negative electric charge found thus far in nature. Beta particles emerge from radioactive material at high speeds, sometimes close to the speed of light.

γ particle   also known as gamma rays, gamma radiation; the most penetrating of all radiations. Gamma rays are very high energy X rays.

X rays   highly penetrating radiation similar to gamma rays. Unlike gamma rays, X rays do not come from the nucleus of the atom but from the surrounding electrons. They are produced by electron bombardment.

μ   micron (equal to approximately 1/25,000 of an inch)

Resource 1:

Union Safety & Health Personnel

AFL-CIO Dept. of Occupational Safety,
Health and Social Security
815 16th St., N.W.
Washington, D.C. 20006
(202) 637-5366
Margaret Seminario, Associate Director

AFL-CIO Building and Construction
Trades Dept.
815 16th St., N.W.
Washington, D.C. 20006
(202) 347-1461
Jim Lapping, Dir., Health & Safety

AFL-CIO Food & Allied Service Trades
815 16th St., N.W.
Washington, D.C. 20006
(202) 737-7200
Debbie Berkowitz, OSHA Program Coord.

AFL-CIO Industrial Union Dept.
815 16th St., N.W.
Washington, D.C. 20006
(202) 842-7800
Sheldon Samuels, Dir., Health,
Safety and Environment

AFL-CIO Metal Trades Dept.
815 16th St., N.W.
Washington, D.C. 20006
(202) 347-7255
Paul Burnsky, President

AFL-CIO Dept. for Professional Employees
815 16th St., N.W.
Washington, D.C. 20006
(202) 638-0320
Dennis Chamot, Asst. Dir.

AFL-CIO Public Employee Dept.
815 16th St., N.W.
Washington, D.C. 20006
(202) 393-2820
Tom Fahey, OSHA Specialist

Air Line Pilots Association
1625 Massachusetts Avenue, N.W.
Washington, D.C. 20036
(202) 797-4188
Joe Schwind, Engineering & Air Safety

Aluminum, Brick and Glass Workers, Int'l
Union
3362 Hollenberg Dr.
Bridgeton, Mo. 63044
(314) 739-6142
L. A. Holley, President

Asbestos Workers, International Assoc. of
Heat and Frost Insulators and
505 Machinists Building
1300 Connecticut Ave., N.W.
Washington, D.C. 20036
(202) 785-2388
Gerald McCarry, Project Director, Health &
Safety Planning

Automobile, Aerospace & Agricultural
Implement Workers, United
Solidarity House
8000 East Jefferson
Detroit, Mich. 48212
(313) 926-5321
Frank Mirer, Director, Health & Safety
Dept.

Bakery, Confectionery and Tobacco Wkrs.
10401 Connecticut Ave.
Kensington, Md. 20895
(301) 933-8600
Vaughn Ball, Dir. of Research and
Education

Boilermakers, Int'l Brotherhood of
570 New Brotherhood Building
8th Street at State Avenue
Kansas City, Kansas 66101
(913) 371-2640
Michael Wood, Dir. of Safety &
Communications

Bricklayers and Allied Craftsmen
815 15th St., N.W.
Washington, D.C. 20005
(202) 783-3788
Merlin Taylor, Director of Safety

Bridge, Structural & Ornamental Iron
Workers
1750 New York Ave., N.W., Suite 400
Washington, D.C. 20006
(202) 383-4800
Robert P. Cooney, Nat'l Safety Chairman

Carpenters, United Brotherhood of
101 Constitution Ave., N.W.
Washington, D.C. 20001
(202) 546-6206
Nicholas R. Loope, Dir., Research, Safety
& Health

Cement, Lime, Gypsum & Allied Workers
Div. of Int'l Bro. of Boilermakers
2500 Brickvale Drive
Elk Grove Village, Ill. 60007
(312) 595-5171
Bill Kojola, Dir. of Safety & Health

Chemical Workers Union, International
1655 W. Market Street
Akron, Ohio 44313
(216) 867-2444
Dave Ortlieb, Director of Health and Safety

Clothing & Textile Wkrs, Amalgamated
15 Union Square
New York, N.Y. 10003
(212) 242-0700
Eric Frumin, Dir., Health & Safety Dept.

Communications Workers of America
1925 K Street, N.W.
Washington, D.C. 20006
(202) 728-2300
David E. LeGrande, Safety & Health Rep.

Electrical, Radio & Machine Workers of
America, United
11 E. 51st St.
New York, N.Y. 10022
(212) 753-1960
David Kotelchuck, Safety and Health Dir.

Electrical Workers, Int'l Brotherhood of
1125 15th Street, N.W.
Washington, D.C. 20005
(202) 833-6137
George Smith, Dir. of Safety

Electronic, Electrical, Technical, Salaried
and Machine Workers, Int'l Union of
1126 16th St., N.W.
Washington, D.C. 20036
(202) 296-1200
Janie Gordon, Health & Safety Dir.

Farm Workers of America, United
P.O. Box 62
Keene, Calif. 93531
(805) 822-5571
Cesar E. Chavez, President

Fire Fighters, Int'l Assn. of
United Unions Building
1750 New York Ave., N.W.
Washington, D.C. 20006
(202) 872-8484
Mike Smith, Dir. of Research
Richard Duffy, Safety and Health
Coordinator

Firemen and Oilers, Int'l Brotherhood of
V.F.W. Bldg., 5th Floor
200 Maryland Ave., N.E.
Washington, D.C. 20002
(202) 737-5300

Flight Attendants, Assn. of
1625 Massachusetts Ave., N.W.
Washington, D.C. 20036
(202) 328-5400
Matthew Finucan, Director of Safety

Food and Commercial Workers, United
1775 K St., N.W.
Washington, D.C. 20006
(202) 223-3111
Jean Giuliana, OSHA Coordinator

Furniture Workers of America, United
1910 Airlane Drive, P.O. Box 100037
Nashville, Tenn. 37210
(615) 889-8860
Lowell Daily, OSHA Director

Garment Workers of America, United
200 Park Ave., South
New York, N.Y. 10003
(212) 677-0573
William O'Donnell, President

Garment Workers Union, Int'l Ladies'
1710 Broadway
New York, New York 10019
(212) 265-7000
Joseph Danahy, Director,
Organization and Field Services

Glass, Pottery, Plastics and Allied Wkrs.
608 E. Baltimore Pike
Media, Pa. 19063
(215) 565-5051
Gilbert Shepherd, Jr., Dir. of Organization
Myran C. Reed, Dir. of Research &
Education

Glass Workers Union, American Flint
1440 S. Byrne Rd.
Toledo, Ohio 43614
(419) 385-6687
Lawrence Bankowski, Asst. Secy.

Government Employees, American Fed. of
1325 Mass. Ave., N.W.
Washington, D.C. 20005
(202) 737-8700 Ext. 259
John Albertson, Safety Specialist
Neil Davis, Industrial Hygienist

Grain Millers, American Fed. of
4949 Olson Memorial Highway
Minneapolis, Minn. 55422
(612) 545-0211
Larry Jackson, Sec.-Treas.

Graphic Communications Int'l Union
1900 L Street, N.W.
Washington, D.C. 20036
(202) 872-7928
Jack Kain, Dir. of Safety and Health

Hotel Employees & Restaurant Employees
1219 28th St., N.W.
Washington, D.C. 20007
Edward T. Hanley, President

Industrial Workers, Allied
3520 West Oklahoma Avenue
Milwaukee, Wis. 53215
(414) 645-9500
Ray MacDonald, Research Dir.
Milan Racic, Dir., Health & Safety

Laborers' International Union
905 16th Street, N.W.
Washington, D.C. 20006
(202) 737-8320
Joe M. Short, Dir. of Education and
Training

Letter Carriers, Nat'l Assn. of
100 Indiana Ave., N.W.
Washington, D.C. 20001
(202) 393-4695
Joseph H. Johnson, Dir., City Delivery

Locomotive Engineers, Bro. of
1112 Bro. of Locomotive Engineers
Building
Cleveland, Ohio 44114
(216) 241-2630
Jan Young, Health & Welfare Director

Longshoremen's Ass'n, International
17 Battery Place, Room 1530
New York, New York 10004
(212) 425-1200
Joseph Leonard, Safety Dir.

Longshoremen's & Warehousemen's
Union, Int'l
1188 Franklin St.
San Francisco, Calif. 94109
(415) 775-0533
Russell Bargmann, Health and Safety
Coordinator

Machinists and Aerospace Wkrs, Int'l
Ass'n of
Machinists Building
1300 Connecticut Avenue, N.W.
Washington, D.C. 20036
(202) 857-5200
George Robinson, Dir. of Occupational
Safety & Health

Maintenance of Way Employees,
Brotherhood of
12050 Woodward Ave.
Detroit, Mich. 48203
(313) 868-0489
Ole M. Berge, President

Marine & Shipbuilding Workers of
America, Industrial Union of
8121 Georgia Ave., Suite 700
Silver Spring, Md. 20910
(301) 589-8820

Marine Engineers' Beneficial Assn.,
National
444 N. Capitol St., Suite 800
Washington, D.C. 20001
(202) 347-8585
Maria Liptak, Asst. to President
Frank Laurito, Treasurer

Maritime Union of America, Nat'l.
346 W. 17th St.
New York, N.Y. 10011
(212) 620-5700
Al Zeidel, Safety Director

Mechanics Educational Society of America
15300 East Seven Mile Rd.
Detroit, Mich. 48205
(313) 372-5700

Mine Workers of America, United
900 15th Street, N.W.
Washington, D.C. 20005
(202) 842-7290
Dr. Lorin E. Kerr, Dir.
of Occupational Health

Molders and Allied Workers Union
1225 E. McMillan Street
Cincinnati, Ohio 45206
(513) 221-1525
Jim Wolfe, Dir. of Education and Research

National Education Assn.
1201 - 16th St., N.W.
Washington, D.C. 20036
Communications Services

Newspaper Guild, The
1125 15th St., N.W.
Washington, D.C. 20005
(202) 296-2990
David J. Eisen, Research Director

Nurses' Association, American
2420 Pershing Rd.
Kansas City, Mo. 64108
(816) 474-5720
Larry Stacy, Dir. of Human Resources

Office & Professional Employees Int'l
Union
265 W. 14th St., Suite 610
New York, N.Y. 10011
(212) 675-3210
Gwen Wells, Research Director

Oil, Chemical and Atomic Workers
225 Union Blvd.
Lakewood, Colorado 80228
(303) 987-2229
Dan Edwards, Health & Safety Dir.

Operating Engineers, Int'l Union of
1125 17th Street, N.W.
Washington, D.C. 20036
(202) 429-9100
Ben Hill, Dir. of Health & Safety

Painters and Allied Trades, Int'l
Brotherhood of
United Unions Building
1750 New York Avenue, N.W.
Washington, D.C. 20006
(202) 637-0700
Rod Wolford
Health and Safety Dir.

Paperworkers International Union, United
702 Church St., P.O. Box 1475
Nashville, Tenn. 37202
(615) 254-6666
Robert R. Frase
Dir. of Occupational Safety and Health

Plasterers' and Cement Masons' Int'l Assn.
1125 17th Street, N.W.
Washington, D.C. 20036
(202) 393-6569
Keith Bell
Coordinator, Safety and Health Program

Plumbers & Pipe Fitters
(United Association)
901 Massachusetts Avenue, N.W.
Washington, D.C. 20001
(202) 628-5823
Joe Adam, Director, Safety Dept.

Postal Workers Union, American
817 14th St., N.W.
Washington, D.C. 20005
(202) 842-4200
Gerald Anderson, Asst. Dir., Clerk Division

Railway, Airline & Steamship
Clerks, Freight Handlers, Express &
Station Employes, Brotherhood of
3 Research Place
Rockville, Md. 20850
(301) 948-4910
R.I. Kilroy, President

Railway Carmen, Brotherhood of
4929 Main St., Carmen's Bldg.
Kansas City, Mo. 64112
(816) 561-1112
Orville W. Jacobson, President

Retail, Wholesale & Dept. Store Union
30 E. 29th St., 4th flr.
New York, N.Y. 10016
(212) 684-5300
Alvin E. Heaps, President

Roofers, Waterproofers and Allied Workers
1125 17th Street, N.W.
Washington, D.C. 20036
(202) 638-2541
John Barnhard, Occupational Safety &
Health Specialist

Rubber, Cork, Linoleum and Plastic
Workers, United
URWA Building
87 S. High Street
Akron, Ohio 44308
(216) 376-6181
Louis Beliczky, Dir. of Industrial Hygiene

Seafarers International Union
5201 Auth Way & Britannia Way
Camp Springs, Md. 20746
(301) 899-0675
Bob Vahey, Safety & Health Dir.

Service Employees Int'l Union
2020 K St., N.W.
Washington, D.C. 20006
(202) 452-8750
Leo Borwegen, OSH Program Coordinator

Sheet Metal Workers
1750 New York Avenue, N.W.
Washington, D.C. 20006
(202) 783-5880
Ralph Wilham
Dir. of Governmental Affairs

Signalmen, Brotherhood of Railroad
601 W. Golf Rd.
Mount Prospect, Ill. 60056
(312) 439-3732
R. T. Bates, President

State, County & Municipal Employees,
American Fed. of
1625 L Street, N.W.
Washington, D.C. 20036
(202) 429-1000
Don Wasserman
Dir. of Research & Collective Bargaining
Services

Steelworkers of America, United
Five Gateway Center
Pittsburgh, Pa. 15222
(412) 562-2581
Frank Grimes
Dir. of Safety & Health Department
Michael Wright, Industrial Hygienist

Teachers, American Federation of
555 New Jersey Ave., N.W.
Washington, D.C. 20001
(202) 879-4458

Teamsters, Int'l Brotherhood of
25 Louisiana Avenue, N.W.
Washington, D.C. 20001
(202) 624-6960
R. V. Durham, Dir. of Safety & Health
Dept.
Suzanne Kossan, Industrial Hygienist

Textile Workers of America, United
420 Common St.
Lawrence, Mass. 01840
(617) 686-2901
Francis Schaufenbil, President

Train Dispatchers Association, American
1401 S. Harlem Ave.
Berwyn, Ill. 60402
(312) 795-5656
R. E. Johnson, President

Transit Union, Amalgamated
5025 Wisconsin Ave., N.W.
Washington, D.C. 20016
(202) 537-1645
Joseph Jaquay, Dir. of Research

Transport Workers Union of America
1980 Broadway
New York, N.Y. 10023
(212) 873-6000
Wm. Kirrane, International Vice President
& Dir. of Education

Transportation Union, United
400 First St., N.W.
Washington, D.C. 20001
(202) 783-3939
James R. Snyder, Legislative Dir.

Typographical Union, Int'l
301 S. Union Blvd., PO Box 157
Colorado Springs, Colo. 80901
(303) 636-2341
Horst A. Reschke
Director, Union Label & Public Relations
Bureau

Utility Workers Union of America
815-16th St., N.W. Ste. 605
Washington, D.C. 20006
(202) 347-8105
Marshall Hicks, Safety & Health Dir.
Michael Kenny, Asst. Dir.

Woodworkers of America, Int'l
1622 N. Lombard Street
Portland, Oregon 97217
(503) 285-5281
R. Denny Scott, Research Economist

Resource 2:

Local & State COSH Groups

COSH stands for Committee or Coalition or Council on Occupational Safety and Health. COSH groups have been formed by workers and health activists concerned about workplace safety and health. They are funded by unions, membership dues, grants and foundations. They rely on volunteers, union staffers, physicians, nurses, occupational hygienists, chemists, lawyers, educators and students. COSH groups have provided training and educational sessions for union locals, set up screening clinics, researched toxic substances and offered expert testimony at government hearings.

The following list was provided by the national COSH coordinators at PHILA-POSH in Philadelphia and the UAW Health and Safety Department.

CALIFORNIA
Santa Clara Center (SCCOSH) for Occupational Safety & Health
361 Willow Street #3
San Jose, Calif., 95110
(408) 998-4050

San Diego (COSH)
3052 Clairemont Street — Ste. 8
San Diego, Calif. 92117
(714) 275-2440

White Lung Association
P.O. Box 5089
San Pedro, Calif. 90733
(213) 832-5864

LACOSH
724 S. Parkview
Los Angeles, Calif. 90057
(213) 387-7281

Bay Area (COSH)
5250 Desmond
Oakland, Calif. 94618
(415) 655-2383

CONNECTICUT
ConnectiCOSH
c/o IAM Local 2746-A
1228 Queen Street
Southington, Conn. 04689

ILLINOIS
Chicago Area COSH (CACOSH)
542 South Dearborn, #502
Chicago, Ill. 60605
(312) 939-2104

Central Illinois (CICOSH)
c/o UAW Local 974
200 East Globe Street
East Peoria, Ill. 61611
(309) 694-3151

KENTUCKY
National Black Lung Assoc.
P.O. Box 187
Harlan, Kentucky 40831

MARYLAND
MaryCOSH
305 West Monument St.
Baltimore, Maryland 21201
(301) 837-0414

MASSACHUSETTS
MassCOSH
718 Huntington Ave.
Boston, Mass. 02115
(617) 277-0097

MassCOSH (Western Region)
458 Bridge Street
Springfield, Mass. 01103
(413) 732-2847

MICHIGAN
Southeast Michigan Coalition on Occup. Safety & Health (SEMCOSH)
1550 Howard
Detroit, Mich. 48216
(313) 961-3345

Michigan RTK Task Force
P.O. Box 24142
Lansing, Mich. 48909
(517) 355-7673

NEW JERSEY
Metro Newark COSH (NJCOSH)
103 Washington Street
Newark, N.J. 07102
(201) 964-0470

New Jersey RTK Coalition South Jersey Committee
911 Billingsport Road
Gibbstown, N.J. 08027
(609) 423-3615

NEW YORK
NYCOSH
32 Union Square #404
New York,, N.Y. 10003
(212) 674-1595

Central New York (CNYCOSH)
615 West Genessee Street
Syracuse, N.Y. 13204
(315) 422-5184

New York State COSH (NYCOSH)
c/o John Becger
1406 Dodge Road
Getzville, N.Y. 14068
(716) 634-3540

Allegheny COSH (ALCOSH)
c/o IBEW Local 1124
45 Maltby Street
Jamestown, N.Y. 14701
(716) 484-1280

Western New York (WNYCOSH)
529 Franklin Street
Buffalo, N.Y. 14202
(716) 886-5546/886-5545

ENYCOSH
Eastern New York COSH
P.O. Box 1618
Albany, N.Y. 12201
(518) 271-8385

ROCOSH — Rochester COSH
c/o Pres. IUE — Local #323
474 Thurston Road
Rochester, N.Y. 14619
(716) 436-2020

Oneida-Herkimer COSH (OHCOSH)
c/o CSEA
314 South Bellenger Street
Herkimer, N.Y. 12250
(315) 735-6101

NORTH CAROLINA
NCOSH
P.O. Box 2514
Durham, N.C. 27705
(919) 286-9249

**Brown Lung Association Greensboro
Chapter**
P.O. Box 13296
Greensboro, N.C. 27405

OHIO
Northeast Ohio COSH NEOCOSH
1793 Wilton Road
Cleveland, Heights, Ohio 44118

Ohio River Valley COSH (ORVCOSH)
2121 Bennett Avenue
Cincinnati, Ohio 45212
(513) 221-1605

WICH of Toledo
c/o Dale Stromer
AFL-CIO Council
320 West Woodruff Avenue
Toledo, Ohio 43624

Youngstown-Warren COSH
Tom Letson, Chairperson
c/o Copperweld USWA Local 2234
Warren, Ohio 44483

COCOSH
1187 East Broad — Suite 21
Columbus, Ohio 43205

OHIO COSH
c/o Ohio AFL-CIO
271 East State Street
Columbus, Ohio 43215
(614) 224-8271

W.I.C.H.S. of Akron/Canton
c/o Kevin Haverfield
IBEW Local 1985
111 S. Main Street
North Canton, Ohio 44720

PENNSYLVANIA
**Western Penn. Comm. for Worker
Safety & Health**
P.O. Box 4951
Pittsburgh, Pa. 15206
(412) 339-8670

**Philaposh Philadelphia Area Project
on Occup. Safety & Health**
3001 Walnut — 5th Floor
Philadelphia, Pa. 19104
(215) 386-7000

RHODE ISLAND
RICOSH
340 Lockwood St.
Providence, R.I. 02907
(401) 751-2015

SOUTH CAROLINA
**Brown Lung Association Greenville
Chapter**
P.O. Box 334
Greenville, S.C. 29602
(803) 269-8229

TENNESSEE
Tennessee COSH (TNCOSH)
Flat Iron Bldg. Room 212
705 N. Broadway
Knoxville, Tenn. 37917
(615) 525-3147

WASHINGTON
SEACOSH
P.O. Box 22636
Seattle, Wash. 98122
(206) 329-8195
(206) 722-5241

WASHINGTON, D.C.
Washington Area COSH
c/o Urban Environ. Conference
815 - 16th St., N.W. Rm 706
Washington, D.C. 20006
(202) 638-6929

WEST VIRGINIA
Kanawah Valley COSH (KVCOSH)
Box 5202
Charleston, W.Va. 25331

WISCONSIN
Wisconsin COSH (WISCOSH)
1334 S. 11th Street
Milwaukee, Wis. 53204
(414) 643-0928

CANADA
Windsor OSH Council
824 Tecumseh Rd. East
Windsor, Ontario N8X 2S3

Resource 3:

Occupational Health Clinics

Finding a doctor trained in detecting work-related illnesses can be an obstacle in many areas. But a number of cities now have occupational health clinics staffed with professional personnel. Some have the direct support of central labor councils or local unions.

The services provided by the clinics vary, but often include the following:

• Tests on individuals to detect illness; such tests include lung function exams, hearing exams and blood tests.

• Screening tests on large groups of workers who work at the same place or do the same kind of work to determine whether health problems are job-related.

• Advice on how job hazards can be controlled, or referral to experts.

• Advice on workers' compensation and other legal rights, or referral to experienced lawyers.

• Medical testimony in workers' compensation cases.

The following list was compiled by the American Labor Education Center, 1835 Kilbourne Pl., N.W., Washington, D.C. 20010 and published in its bimonthly newsletter, American Labor. Many clinics have been established in recent years, so if no clinic is listed in your area, check with your union or local COSH group or with universities.

CALIFORNIA
Occupational Health Clinic
San Francisco General Hospital
1001 Potrero Avenue
San Francisco, Calif. 94110
Phone: (415) 821-5391

Barlow-U.S.C. Occupational Health Center
200 Stadium Way
Los Angeles, Calif. 90026
Phone: (213) 250-4200

CONNECTICUT
Yale Occupational Medicine Program
333 Cedar Street
New Haven, Conn. 06510
Phone: (203) 785-4197

ILLINOIS
Occupational Medicine Clinic
Cook County Hospital
720 S. Wolcott
Chicago, Ill. 60612
Phone: (312) 633-5310

KENTUCKY
University of Kentucky Medical Center — Pulmonary Division
800 Rose Street
Lexington, Ky. 40536
Phone: (606) 233-5419

LOUISIANA
Ochner Clinic
Riverfront Center for Occupational Medicine & Environmental Health
625 Jackson Avenue
New Orleans, La. 70130
Phone: (504) 587-0302

MARYLAND
Occupational Medicine Clinic
Baltimore City Hospital
4940 Eastern Avenue
Baltimore, Md. 21224
Phone: (301) 396-8058

MASSACHUSETTS

Occupational Health Clinic
Norfolk County Hospital
2001 Washington Street
So. Braintree, Mass. 02184
Phone: (617) 843-0690

Occupational Health and Environmental Health Center
Brigham and Women's Hospital
721 Huntington Avenue
Boston, Mass. 02115
Phone: (617) 732-5983

Occupational Medicine Clinic
Mass. General Hospital
Fruite Street
Boston, Mass. 02146
Phone: (617) 726-3741/726-2721

Occupational Health Service Department of Family and Community Medicine
University of Mass. Medical Center
55 Lake Avenue North
Worcester, Mass. 01605
Phone: (617) 856-3759

Occupational Medicine Clinic
Cambridge Hospital
1493 Cambridge St.
Cambridge, Mass. 02139
Phone: (617) 498-1024

MICHIGAN

University of Michigan Occupational Health Clinic
School of Public Health II
Room M-6012
Ann Arbor, Mich. 48106
Phone: (313) 763-5174/764-2594

NEW JERSEY

Occupational Medicine Group
714 Broadway
Paterson, N.J. 07514
Phone: (617) 684-5077

Occupational/Environmental Disease Clinic
New Jersey Department of Health
CN-360
Trenton, N.J. 08625
Phone: (609) 984-1863

NEW MEXICO

New Mexico Occupational Health Program
Family Practice/Psych. Bldg.
University of New Mexico School of Medicine
Albuquerque, N.Mex. 87131
Phone: (505) 277-3253

NEW YORK

Mt. Sinai Medical Center
Occupational Medicine Clinic
100th Street & 5th Avenue
New York, N.Y. 10029
Phone: (212) 650-6174

Occupational Health Clinic
Montefiore Hospital
111 E. 210th Street
Bronx, N.Y. 10467
Phone: (212) 920-4766

OHIO

Occupational Health Clinic Department of Environmental Health at Kettering
J-4 Pavilion (4th Floor)
234 Goodman Street
Cincinnati, Ohio 45267
Phone: (513) 872-5284

Cleveland Clinic
9500 Euclid Avenue
Cleveland, Ohio 44106
Phone: (216) 444-2000

TENNESSEE

Knoxville Neighborhood Health Services
1953 Goins Drive
Knoxville, Tenn. 37917
Phone: (615) 546-4606

Center for Health Services
Vanderbilt University
Nashville, Tenn. 37232
Phone: (615) 322-4799

WASHINGTON

Occupational Medicine Clinic
Harborview Medical Center
325 9th Avenue
Seattle, Wash. 98104
Phone: (206) 223-3005

WISCONSIN

Medical College of Wisconsin
Dept. of Preventive Medicine
8701 Watertown Plank Road
Milwaukee, Wis. 53226
Phone: (414) 257-8288

Marshfield Clinic
1000 N. Oak
Marshfield, Wis. 54449
Phone: (715) 387-1713

Clinical Science Center
University Hospital
600 Highland Avenue
Madison, Wis. 53792
Phone: (608) 263-3612

Medical/Surgical Clinic
2400 W. Lincoln Avenue
Milwaukee, Wis. 53215
Phone: (414) 671-7000

CANADA
Hamilton Workers' Clinic
1071 Barton Street, East
Hamilton, Ontario L8L 3E2
Phone: (416) 544-5181

Manitoba Federation of Labour
Occupational Health Centre
98 Sherbrook St.
Winnipeg, Manitoba
Phone: (204) 786-5881

Resource 4:

Allied Organizations

American Cancer Society
777 Third Ave.
New York, N.Y. 10017

American Labor Education Center
1835 Kilbourne Pl., N.W.
Washington, D.C. 20010
(202) 387-6780

American Lung Association
1740 Broadway
New York, N.Y. 10019
(212) 245-8000

American Public Health Association
1015 15th St., N.W.
Washington, D.C. 20005
(202) 789-5600

Coalition for Labor Union Women
(CLUW)
Center for Education and Research
2000 P St., N.W. Room 615
Washington, D.C. 20036
(202) 296-3408

Collegium Ramazzini
P.O. Box 50
Solomons, Md. 20688
(202) 842-7833

Environmental Action Foundation
724 Dupont Circle Building
Washington, D.C. 20036
(202) 296-7570

Environmentalists for Full Employment
1536 16th St., N.W.
Washington, D.C. 20036
(202) 347-5590

Health Research Group
2000 P St., N.W. Room 708
Washington, D.C. 20036
(202) 872-0320

Labor Occupational Health Program
(LOHP)
Institute of Industrial Relations,
Center for Labor Research and Education
University of California
2521 Channing Way
Berkeley, Calif. 94720
(415) 642-5507

National Safety Council
444 N. Michigan Avenue
Chicago, Illinois 60611
(312) 527-4800

Natural Resources Defense Council
122 E. 42nd St.
New York, N.Y. 10168
(212) 949-0094

9 to 5 National Association
1224 Huron Rd.
Cleveland, Ohio 44115
(216) 566-9308

Sierra Club
530 Bush St.
San Francisco, Calif. 94108
(415) 981-8634

Society for Occupational and Environmental Health
2021 K St., N.W.
Washington, D.C. 20006
(202) 737-5045

Urban Environment Conference
815 - 16th St., N.W. Rm 706
Washington, D.C. 20006
(202) 638-6929

Western Institute for Occupational and Environmental Sciences, Inc.
2520 Milvia
Berkeley, Calif. 94704
(415) 845-6476

Women's Occupational Health Resource Center
Columbia University School of Public Health
60 Haven Ave., B-1
New York, N.Y. 10032
(212) 694-3737

Workers' Institute for Safety & Health
1126 - 16th St., N.W.
Washington, D.C. 20036
(202) 887-1980

Workplace Health Fund
815 - 16th St., N.W.
Washington, D.C. 20006
(202) 842-7833

Resource 5:

U.S. Department of Labor Occupational Safety & Health Admin.

Directory of Field Locations

BOSTON — REGION I Connecticut, Maine, Massachusetts, New Hampshire, Rhode Island and Vermont

BOSTON REGIONAL OFFICE
Regional Administrator
US Department of Labor — OSHA
16-18 North Street
1 Dock Square Building 4th Floor
Boston, Massachusetts 02109
(617) 223-6710

Boston Area Office
US Department of Labor - OSHA
400-2 Totten Pond Road 2nd Floor
Waltham, Massachusetts 02154
(617) 647-8681

Concord Area Office
US Department of Labor - OSHA
Federal Building Rm. 334
55 Pleasant Street
Concord, New Hampshire 03301
(603) 224-1995

Providence Area Office
US Department of Labor - OSHA
380 Westminster Mall - Rm. 243
Providence, Rhode Island 02903
(401) 528-4669

Springfield Area Office
US Department of Labor - OSHA
1550 Main Street Rm. 532
Springfield, Massachusetts 01103-01493
(413) 785-0123

Augusta Area Office
US Department of Labor - OSHA
40 Western Avenue Rm. 121
Augusta, Maine 04330
(207) 622-8417 Ext. 417

Hartford Area Office
US Department of Labor - OSHA
Federal Office Bldg.
450 Main Street - Rm. 508
Hartford, Connecticut 06103
(203) 244-2294

NEW YORK CITY — REGION II New Jersey, New York and Puerto Rico

NEW YORK REGIONAL OFFICE
Regional Administrator
US Department of Labor - OSHA
1515 Broadway (1 Astor Plaza) Rm. 3445
New York, New York 10036
(212) 944-3432

Manhattan Area Office — Vacant

Long Island Area Office
US Department of Labor - OSHA
990 Westbury Road
Westbury, New York 11590
(516) 334-3344

Queens Area Office
US Department of Labor - OSHA
136-21 Roosevelt Avenue 3rd Floor
Flushing, New York 11354
(212) 445-5005

Albany Area Office
US Department of Labor - OSHA
Leo W. O'Brien Federal Building
Clinton Avenue & North Pearl Street Rm.
132
Albany, New York 12207
(518) 472-6085

Syracuse Area Office
US Department of Labor - OSHA
100 South Clinton Street Rm. 1267
Syracuse, New York 13260
Comm. Phone: (315) 423-5188
FTS Phone: 950-5188

Buffalo Area Office
US Department of Labor - OSHA
220 Delaware Avenue Suite 509
Buffalo, New York 14202
Comm. Phone: (716) 846-4881
FTS Phone: 437-4881

Puerto Rico Area Office
US Department of Labor - OSHA
US Courthouse & FOB
Carlos Chardon Avenue Rm. 555
Hato Rey, Puerto Rico 00918
(809) 753-4457/4072

Hasbrouck Heights Area Office
US Department of Labor - OSHA
Teterboro Airport Professional Building
377 Route 17 Rm. 206
Hasbrouck Heights, New Jersey 07604
(201) 288-1700

Belle Mead Area Office
US Department of Labor - OSHA
Belle Mead GSA Depot Building T3
Belle Mead, New Jersey 08502
(201) 359-2777

Camden Area Office
US Department of Labor - OSHA
2101 Ferry Avenue Rm. 403
Camden, New Jersey 08104
(609) 757-5181

Dover Area Office
US Department of Labor - OSHA
2 East Blackwell Street
Dover, New Jersey 07801
(201) 361-4050

PHILADELPHIA — REGION III Delaware, District of Columbia, Maryland, Pennsylvania, Virginia, and West Virginia

PHILADELPHIA REGIONAL OFFICE
Regional Administrator
US Department of Labor - OSHA
Gateway Building Suite 2100
3535 Market Street
Philadelphia, Pennsylvania 19104
(215) 596-1201

Philadelphia Area Office
US Department of Labor - OSHA
Rm. 242 US Custom House
Second & Chestnut Street
Philadelphia, Pennsylvania 19106
(215) 597-4955

Wilmington District Office
US Department of Labor - OSHA
Federal Office Building Rm. 3007
844 King Street
Wilmington, Delaware 19801
(302) 573-6115

Pittsburgh Area Office
US Department of Labor - OSHA
Federal Building Rm. 2236
1000 Liberty Avenue
Pittsburgh, Pennsylvania 15522
(412) 644-2903

Erie District Office
US Department of Labor - OSHA
147 West 18th Street
Erie, Pennsylvania 16501
(814) 453-4351

Wilkes-Barre Area Office
US Department of Labor - OSHA
Penn Place Rm. 2005
20 North Pennsylvania Avenue
Wilkes-Barre, Pennsylvania 18701
(717) 826-6538

Allentown Office
U.S. Department of Labor - OSHA
850 N. 5th Street
Allentown, Pennsylvania 18102
(215) 776-4220

Charleston Area Office
US Department of Labor - OSHA
500 Eagan Street Rm. 206
Charleston, West Virginia 25301
(304) 347-5937

Harrisburg Area Office
US Department of Labor - OSHA
Progress Plaza
49 North Progress Avenue
Harrisburg, Pennsylvania 17109
(717) 782-3902

Baltimore Area Office
US Department of Labor - OSHA
Federal Building Rm. 1110
Charles Center 31 Hopkins Plaza
Baltimore, Maryland 21201
(301) 962-2840

Richmond District Office
US Department of Labor - OSHA
Federal Building Rm. 6226
400 North 8th Street
PO Box 10186
Richmond, Virginia 23240
(804) 771-2864

ATLANTA — REGION IV Alabama, Florida, Georgia, Kentucky, Mississippi, North Carolina, South Carolina and Tennessee

ATLANTA REGIONAL OFFICE
Regional Administrator
US Department of Labor - OSHA
1375 Peachtree Street, N.E. Suite 587
Atlanta, Georgia 30367
(404) 881-3573

Atlanta Area Office
US Department of Labor - OSHA
Building 10 Suite 33
LaVista Perimeter Office Park
Tucker, Georgia 30084
(404) 221-4767

Savannah District Office
US Department of Labor - OSHA
1600 Drayton Street
Savannah, Georgia 31401
(912) 233-2923

Birmingham Area Office
US Department of Labor - OSHA
Todd Mall
2047 Canyon Road
Birmingham, Alabama 35216
(205) 822-7100

Mobile District Office
US Department of Labor - OSHA
951 Government Street Suite 502
Mobile, Alabama 36604
(205) 690-2131

Columbia Area Office
US Department of Labor - OSHA
1835 Assembly Street Rm. 1468
Columbia, South Carolina 29201
(803) 765-5904

Jackson Area Office
US Department of Labor - OSHA
Federal Building Suite 1445
100 West Capitol Street
Jackson, Mississippi 39269
(601) 960-4606

Fort Lauderdale Area Office
US Department of Labor - OSHA
Federal Building Room 302
299 East Broward Boulevard
Fort Lauderdale, Florida 33301
(305) 527-7292

Jacksonville Area Office
US Department of Labor - OSHA
Art Museum Plaza Suite 17
2747 Art Museum Drive
Jacksonville, Florida 32207
(904) 791-2895

Tampa Area Office
US Department of Labor - OSHA
700 Twiggs Street Room 624
Tampa, Florida 33602
(813) 228-2821

Nashville Area Office
US Department of Labor - OSHA
1720 West End Ave. Suite 302
Nashville, Tennessee 37203
(615) 251-5313

Frankfort Area Office — Vacant

Raleigh Area Office
US Department of Labor - OSHA
Federal Office Building Room 406
310 New Bern Avenue
Raleigh, North Carolina 27601
(919) 755-4770

CHICAGO — REGION V Indiana, Illinois, Michigan, Minnesota, Ohio and Wisconsin

CHICAGO REGIONAL OFFICE
Regional Administrator
US Department of Labor - OSHA
32nd Floor Rm. 3244
230 South Dearborn Street
Chicago, Illinois 60604
(312) 353-2220

Calumet City Area Office
US Department of Labor - OSHA
1400 Torrence Avenue - 2nd Floor
Calumet City, Illinois 60409
(312) 891-3800

Niles Area Office
US Department of Labor - OSHA
6000 West Touhy Avenue
Niles, Illinois 60648
(312) 631-8200/8535

Aurora Area Office
US Department of Labor - OSHA
344 Smoke Tree Business Park
North Aurora, Illinois 60542
(312) 896-8700

Cincinnati Area Office
US Department of Labor - OSHA
Federal Office Building Rm. 4028
550 Main Street
Cincinnati, Ohio 45202
(513) 684-3784

Cleveland Area Office
US Department of Labor - OSHA
Federal Office Building Rm. 899
1240 East 9th Street
Cleveland, Ohio 44199
(216) 522-3818

Columbus Area Office
US Department of Labor - OSHA
Federal Office Building Rm. 634
200 North High Street
Columbus, Ohio 43215
(614) 469-5582

Indianapolis Area Office
US Department of Labor - OSHA
USPO & Courthouse Rm. 422
46 East Ohio Street
Indianapolis, Indiana 46204
(317) 269-7290

Appleton Area Office
US Department of Labor - OSHA
2618 North Ballard Road
Appleton, Wisconsin 54915
(414) 734-4521

Eau Claire District Office
US Department of Labor - OSHA
Federal Building US Courthouse
500 Barstow Street Rm. B-9
Eau Claire, Wisconsin 54701
(715) 832-9019

Milwaukee Area Office
US Department of Labor - OSHA
Henry S. Reuss Bldg.
310 Wisconsin Ave, Suite 1180
Milwaukee, Wisconsin 53203
(414) 291-3315

Madison District Office
US Department of Labor - OSHA
2934 Fish Hatchery Road Suite 220
Madison, Wisconsin 53713
(608) 264-5388

Toledo Area Office
US Department of Labor - OSHA
Federal Office Building Rm. 734
234 North Summit Street
Toledo, Ohio 43604
(419) 259-7542

Minneapolis Area Office
US Department of Labor - OSHA
801 Butler Square Building
100 North 6th Street
Minneapolis, Minnesota 55403
(612) 725-2571

Peoria Area Office
US Department of Labor - OSHA
3024 West Lake St.
Peoria, Illinois 61615
(309) 671-7033

Belleville District Office
US Department of Labor - OSHA
218A Main Street
Belleville, Illinois 62220
(618) 277-5300

Detroit Area Office
US Department of Labor - OSHA
231 West LaFayette Rm. 628
Detroit, Michigan 48226
(313) 226-6720

DALLAS — REGION VI Arkansas, Louisiana, New Mexico, Oklahoma and Texas

DALLAS REGIONAL OFFICE
Regional Administrator
US Department of Labor - OSHA
555 Griffin Square Building Rm. 602
Dallas, Texas 75202
(214) 767-4731

Dallas Area Office
US Department of Labor - OSHA
1425 West Pioneer Drive
Irving, Texas, 75061
(214) 767-5347

Albuquerque Area Office
US Department of Labor - OSHA
Western Bank Building Rm. 1407
505 Marquette Avenue, N.W.
Albuquerque, New Mexico 87102
(505) 776-3411

Corpus Christi Area Office
US Department of Labor - OSHA
4455 S. Padre Drive Suite 50
Corpus Christi, Texas 78411
(512) 888-3257

Austin Area Office
US Department of Labor - OSHA
303 Grant Bldg.
611 East 6th Street
Austin, Texas 78701
(512) 482-5783

Baton Rouge Area Office
US Department of Labor - OSHA
Hoover Annex Suite 200
2156 Wooddale Boulevard
Baton Rouge, Louisiana 70806
(504) 389-0474

Lubbock Area Office
US Department of Labor - OSHA
Federal Building Rm. 421
1205 Texas Avenue
Lubbock, Texas 79401
(806) 743-7681

Houston Area Office
US Department of Labor - OSHA
2320 LaBranch Street Room 1103
Houston, Texas 77004
(713) 750-1727

Little Rock Area Office
US Department of Labor - OSHA
Savers Bldg. Suite 828
320 West Capitol Ave.
Little Rock, Arkansas 72201
(501) 378-6291

Oklahoma City Area Office
US Department of Labor - OSHA
50 Penn Place Suite 502
Oklahoma City, Oklahoma 73118
(405) 231-5351

KANSAS CITY — REGION VII Iowa, Kansas, Missouri and Nebraska

KANSAS CITY REGIONAL OFFICE
Regional Administrator
US Department of Labor - OSHA
911 Walnut Street Rm. 406
Kansas City, Missouri 64106
(816) 374-5861

Kansas City Area Office
US Department of Labor - OSHA
1150 Grand Avenue 6th Floor
Rm. 606
Kansas City, Missouri 64106
(816) 374-2756

Des Moines Area Office
US Department of Labor - OSHA
210 Walnut Street Rm. 815
Des Moines, Iowa 50309
(515) 284-4794

Omaha Area Office
US Department of Labor - OSHA
Overland - Wolf Building Rm. 100
6910 Pacific Street
Omaha, Nebraska 68106
(402) 221-3182

St. Louis Area Office
US Department of Labor - OSHA
4300 Goodfellow Boulevard
Building 105E
St. Louis, Missouri 63120
(314) 263-2749

Wichita Area Office
US Department of Labor - OSHA
216 North Waco Suite B
Wichita, Kansas 67202
(316) 269-6644

DENVER — REGION VIII Colorado, Montana, North Dakota, South Dakota, Utah and Wyoming

DENVER REGIONAL OFFICE
Regional Administrator
US Department of Labor - OSHA
Federal Building Rm. 1554
1961 Stout Street
Denver Colorado 80294
(303) 837-3061

Billings Area Office
US Department of Labor - OSHA
Petroleum Building Suite 210
2812 1st Avenue North
Billings, Montana 59101
(406) 657-6649

Bismarck Area Office
US Department of Labor - OSHA
Federal Building Rm. 348
PO Box 2439
Bismarck, North Dakota 58501
(701) 255-4011 Ext. 521

Denver Area Office
US Department of Labor - OSHA
Tremont Center - 1st Floor
333 West Colfax
Denver, Colorado 80204
(303) 837-5285

Salt Lake City Area Office
US Department of Labor - OSHA
US Post Office Building - Rm. 505
350 South Main Street
Salt Lake City, Utah 84101
(801) 524-5080

SAN FRANCISCO — REGION IX American Samoa, Arizona, California, Guam, Hawaii, Nevada, Trust Territory of the Pacific Islands

SAN FRANCISCO REGIONAL OFFICE
Regional Administrator
US Department of Labor - OSHA
11349 General Building
450 Golden Gate Avenue
PO Box 36017
San Francisco, California 94102
Comm. Phone: (415) 556-7260

California Area Office
US Department of Labor - OSHA
1960 Addison St, Suite 290
Berkeley, California 94704
(415) 486-3410

Long Beach District Office
US Department of Labor - OSHA
400 Oceangate Suite 530
Long Beach, California 90802
(213) 432-3434

Carson City Area Office
US Department of Labor - OSHA
1050 East William Street Suite 402
Carson City, Nevada 89701
(702) 883-1226

Phoenix Area Office
US Department of Labor - OSHA
Amerco Towers Suite 300
2721 North Central Avenue
Phoenix, Arizona 85004
(602) 241-2007

Honolulu Area Office
US Department of Labor - OSHA
300 Ala Moana Boulevard Suite 5122
PO Box 50072
Honolulu, Hawaii 96850
(808) 546-3157

SEATTLE — REGION X Alaska, Idaho, Oregon and Washington

SEATTLE REGIONAL OFFICE
Regional Administrator
US Department of Labor - OSHA
Federal Office Building Rm. 6003
909 1st Avenue
Seattle, Washington 98174
(206) 442-5930

Anchorage Area Office
US Department of Labor - OSHA
Federal Building
701 C Street Box 29
Anchorage, Alaska 99513
(907) 271-5152

Bellevue Area Office
US Department of Labor - OSHA
121 - 107th Street, N.E.
Bellevue, Washington 98004
(206) 442-7520

Boise Area Office
US Department of Labor - OSHA
1315 West Idaho Street
Boise, Idaho 83702
(208) 334-1867

Portland Area Office
US Department of Labor - OSHA
1220 Southwest 3rd Street Rm. 640
Portland, Oregon 97204
(503) 221-2251

OSHA TRANING INSTITUTE
OSHA Training Institute
US Department of Labor
1555 Times Drive
Des Plaines, Illinois 60018
(312) 297-4810

CINCINNATI LABORATORY
OSHA Cincinnati Laboratory
USPO Building Room 108
5th & Walnut Streets
Cincinnati, Ohio 45202
(513) 684-2531

SALT LAKE CITY LABORATORY
SLC Analytical Laboratory
390 Wakara Way Research Park
Salt Lake City, Utah 84108
(801) 524-5287

HEALTH RESPONSE UNIT, SLC
Health Response Unit - OSHA
390 Wakara Way
Salt Lake City, Utah 84108
(801) 524-5896

Resource 6:

States With Approved Safety and Health Plans

ALASKA
Alaska Department of Labor
Post Office Box 1149
Juneau, Alaska 99802
(907) 465-2700

ARIZONA
Division of Occupational Safety and Health
Industrial Commission of Arizona
P.O. Box 19070
Phoenix, Arizona 85005
(602) 255-5795

CALIFORNIA
Secretary of Industrial Relations
525 Golden Gate Avenue
San Francisco, California 94102
(415) 557-3356

CONNECTICUT
Connecticut Department of Labor
200 Folly Brook Boulevard
Wethersfield, Connecticut 06109
(Public Employees Only)
(203) 566-5123

HAWAII
Hawaii Department of Labor and Industrial
Relations
825 Mililani Street
Honolulu, Hawaii 96813
(808) 548-3150

INDIANA
Indiana Division of Labor
1013 State Office Building
100 North Senate Avenue
Indianapolis, Indiana 46204
(317) 232-2663

IOWA
Iowa Bureau of Labor
State House
307 East Seventh Street
Des Moines, Iowa 50319
(515) 281-3447

KENTUCKY
Kentucky Department of Labor
U.S. Highway 127 South
Frankfort, Kentucky 40601
(502) 564-3070

MARYLAND
Maryland Division of Labor and Industry
Department of Licensing and Regulation
501 St. Paul Place
Baltimore, Maryland 21202
(301) 659-4176

MICHIGAN
Michigan Department of Labor
7150 Harris Drive, Box 30015
Lansing, Michigan 48909
(517) 373-9600

Michigan Department of Public Health
3500 North Logan Street, Box 30015
Lansing, Michigan 48909
(517) 373-1320

MINNESOTA
Minnesota Department of Labor and
Industry
444 Lafayette Road
St. Paul, Minnesota 55101
(612) 296-2342

NEVADA
Department of Industrial Relations
Division of Occupational Safety and Health
Capitol Complex
1370 S. Curry Street
Carson City, Nevada 89710
(702) 885-5240

NEW MEXICO
Environmental Improvement Division
Health and Environment Department
P.O. Box 968
1480 St. Francis Drive
Santa Fe, New Mexico 87503
(505) 984-0020

NORTH CAROLINA
North Carolina Department of Labor
4 West Edenton Street
Raleigh, North Carolina 27601
(919) 733-7166

OREGON
Workers' Compensation Department
Labor and Industries Building
Salem, Oregon 97310
(503) 378-3304

PUERTO RICO
Secretary of Labor and Human Resources
Puerto Rico Department of Labor
Prudencio Rivera Martinez Building
505 Munoz Rivera Avenue
Hato Rey, Puerto Rico 00918
(809) 754-2119-22

SOUTH CAROLINA
South Carolina Department of Labor
3600 Forest Drive
P.O. Box 11329
Columbia, South Carolina 29211
(803) 758-2851
       758-3080

TENNESSEE
Tennessee Department of Labor
ATTN: Robert Taylor
501 Union Building
Suite "A" - 2nd Floor
Nashville, Tennessee 37219
(615) 741-2582

UTAH
Utah Industrial Commission
Utah Occupational Safety and Health
160 East 3rd South
P.O. Box 5800
Salt Lake City, Utah 84110-5800
(801) 530-6900

VERMONT
Vermont Department of Labor and
Industry
118 State Street
Montpelier, Vermont 05602
(802) 828-2765

VIRGIN ISLANDS
Commissioner of Labor
Government of Virgin Islands
Box 890
Christiansted
St. Croix, Virgin Islands 00820
(809) 773-1994

VIRGINIA
Virginia Department of Labor and Industry
P.O. Box 12064
Richmond, Virginia 23241-0064
(804) 786-2376

Virginia Department of Health
James Madison Building
109 Governor Street
Richmond, Virginia 23219
(804) 936-4265

WASHINGTON
Washington Department of Labor and
Industries
General Administration Building
Room 334 - AX-31
Olympia, Washington 98504
(206) 753-6307

WYOMING
Department of Occupational Safety and
Health
604 East 25th Street
Cheyenne, Wyoming 82002
(307) 777-7796

Resource 7:

Department of Health & Human Services
Centers for Disease Control
National Institute for Occupational Safety and Health

Regional Offices

I HHS PHS CDC NIOSH, Region I
JFK Federal Bldg., Room 1401
Boston, Mass. 02203
(617) 223-4045/4046

II HHS PHS CDC NIOSH, Region II
26 Federal Plaza, Room 3300
New York, N.Y. 10278
(212) 264-2485

III HHS PHS CDC NIOSH, Region III
P.O. Box 13716
Philadelphia, Pa. 19101
(215) 596-6716

IV HHS PHS CDC NIOSH, Region IV
101 Marietta Tower, Suite 1007
Atlanta, Ga. 30323
(404) 221-2396

V HHS PHS CDC NIOSH, Region V
300 South Wacker Drive
33rd Floor
Chicago, Ill. 60606
(312) 886-3881

VI HHS PHS CDC NIOSH, Region VI
1200 Main Tower Blvd.,
Rm. 1700-A
Dallas, Texas 75202
(214) 767-3916

VII HHS PHS CDC NIOSH, Region VII
601 E. 12th Street
Kansas City, Mo. 64106
(816) 374-3491

VIII HHS PHS CDC NIOSH, Region VIII
1185 Federal Bldg., 1961 Stout St.
Denver, Colo. 80294
(303) 837-6163

IX HHS PHS CDC NIOSH, Region IX
50 United Nations Plaza, Rm 231
San Francisco, Calif. 94102
(415) 556-3781

X HHS PHS CDC NIOSH, Region X
M/S 402
2901 Third Avenue
Seattle, Wash. 98121
(206) 442-0502

Resource 8:

U.S. Department of Labor
Mine Safety & Health Administration
Division of Coal Mine Safety & Health

DISTRICT 1
Penn Place
20 North Pennsylvania Ave.
Wilkes-Barre, Pa. 18701
(717) 826-6321

DISTRICT 2
4800 Forbes Avenue
Pittsburgh, Pa. 15213
(412) 612-4500 ext. 363

Subdistrict Offices:
Monroeville, Pa.
Johnstown, Pa.

DISTRICT 3
5012 Mountaineer Mall
Morgantown, W.Va. 26505
(304) 291-4277

DISTRICT 4
P.O. Box 112
Mount Hope, W.Va. 25880
(304) 877-6405

Subdistrict Offices:
Princeton, W.Va.
Madison, W.Va.

DISTRICT 5
P.O. Box 560
Norton, Va. 24273
(703) 679-0230

Subdistrict Offices:
Richlands, Va.

DISTRICT 6
218 High Street
Pikeville, Ky. 41501
(606) 437-9616

Subdistrict Offices:
Paintsville, Ky.

DISTRICT 7
P.O. Box 572
Barbourville, Ky. 40906
(606) 546-5123

Subdistrict Offices:
Homewood, Ala.
Hazard, Ky.

DISTRICT 8
P.O. Box 418
Vincennes, Ind. 47591
(812) 882-7616

Subdistrict Offices:
Benton, IL
St. Clairsville, Ohio

DISTRICT 9
P.O. Box 25367
Denver, Colo. 80225
(303) 234-2293

Subdistrict Offices:
Price, Utah

DISTRICT 10
P.O. Box 473
Madisonville, Ky. 42431
(502) 821-4180

Subdistrict Offices:
McAlester, Okla.

TECHNICAL SUPPORT DIRECTORY

Bruceton Safety Technology Center
4800 Forbes Ave
Pittsburgh, Pa. 15213
(412) 675-6400

Pittsburgh Health Technology Center
4800 Forbes Avenue
Pittsburgh, Pa. 15213
(412) 621-4500

Denver Safety & Health Technology
Center
P.O. Box 25367
Denver, Colo. 80225

Approval & Certification Center
P.O. Box 251
Industrial Park Boulevard
Triadelphia, W.Va. 26059
(304) 547-0400 Ext. 71

Health & Safety Analysis Center
P.O. Box 25367
Denver, Colo. 80225

Mine Emergency Operations
Hopewell Facility
1200 Airport Road
Aliquippa, Pa. 15001
(412) 378-0561

Special Projects
4800 Forbes Ave.
Pittsburgh, Pa. 15213

Metal & Nonmetal District Offices

NORTHEASTERN DISTRICT

DISTRICT OFFICE
District Manager
4800 Forbes Avenue
Pittsburgh, Pa. 15213
(412) 621-4500

Pittsburgh Subdistrict Office
Subdistrict Manager
4800 Forbes Avenue
Pittsburgh, Pa. 15213
(412) 621-4500

Field Offices:
Pittsburgh, Pa.
Beckley, W. Va.
Charlottesville, Va.
Wyomissing, Pa.

Albany Subdistrict Office
Subdistrict Manager
P.O. Box 1894
U.S. Post Office & Courthouse
Albany, N.Y. 12201
(518) 472-3648, 3649, 3654

Field Offices:
Albany, N.Y.
Dover, N.J.
Geneva, N.Y.
Springfield, Mass.

SOUTHERN DISTRICT

DISTRICT OFFICE
District Manager
228 West Valley Avenue, Room 102
Birmingham, Ala. 35209
(205) 254-1510, 0660, 1507

Birmingham Subdistrict Office
Subdistrict Manager
228 West Valley Avenue, Room 102
Birmingham, Ala. 35209
(205) 254-1510, 0660

Field Offices:
Birmingham, Ala.
Bartow, Fla.
Macon, Ga.
Hato Rey, Puerto Rico

Knoxville Subdistrict Office
Subdistrict Manager
301 West Cumberland Ave., Room 223
Knoxville, Tenn. 37902
(615) 673-4581

Field Offices:
Knoxville, Tenn.
Columbia, S.C.
Franklin, Tenn.
Lexington, Ky.

NORTH CENTRAL DISTRICT

DISTRICT OFFICE
District Manager
228 Federal Building
Duluth, Minn. 55802
(218) 727-6692 ext. 448

Duluth Subdistrict Office
Subdistrict Manager
228 Federal Building
Duluth, Minn. 55802
(218) 727-6692 ext. 451

Field Offices:
Duluth, Minn.
Hibbing, Minn.
Lansing, Mich.
Marquette, Mich.

Vincennes Subdistrict Office
Subdistrict Manager
P.O. Box 927
501 Busseron Street
Vincennes, Ind. 47491
(812) 882-0696

Field Offices:
Vincennes, Ind.
Newark, Ohio
Peru, Ill.

SOUTH CENTRAL DISTRICT

DISTRICT OFFICE
District Manager
1100 Commerce Street, Room 4C50
Dallas, Texas 75242
(214) 767-8401

Dallas Subdistrict Office
Subdistrict Manager
1100 Commerce Street
Dallas, Texas 75242
(214) 767-8402, 8403

Field Offices:
Dallas, Texas
Albuquerque, N.M.
Baton Rouge, La.
Carlsbad, N.M.
Grants, N.M.
Little Rock, Ark.
San Antonio, Texas
Oklahoma City, Okla.

Rolla Subdistrict Office
Subdistrict Manager
P.O. Box 1156 (900 Pine St.)
Rolla, Mo. 65401
(314) 364-8282

Field Offices:
Rolla, Mo.
Omaha, Neb.
Topeka, Kan.

ROCKY MOUNTAIN DISTRICT

DISTRICT OFFICE
District Manager
P.O. Box 25367, DFC
Denver, Colo. 80225
(303) 234-3421

Denver Subdistrict Office
Subdistrict Manager
P.O. Box 25367, DFC
Denver, Colo. 80225
(303) 234-2271

Field Offices:
Denver, Colo.
Grand Junction, Colo.
Rapid City, S.D.

Salt Lake City Subdistrict
Subdistrict Manager
307 West 200 South, Suite 3002,3
Salt Lake City, Utah 84101
(801) 524-5385

Field Offices:
Salt Lake City, Utah
Green River, Wyo.
Helena, Mont.
Moab, Utah
Riverton, Wyo.

WESTERN DISTRICT OFFICE

DISTRICT OFFICE
District Manager
620 Central Avenue, Building 7
Alameda, Calif. 94501
(415) 273-7457, 7011

Bellevue Subdistrict Office
Subdistrict Manager
117 107th Avenue N.E., Room 100
Belevue, Wash. 98004
(206) 422-7037, 5455

Field Offices:
Bellevue, Wash.
Boise, Idaho
Coeur d'Alene, Idaho

Phoenix Subdistrict Office
Subdistrict Manager
2721 N. Central Avenue, Suite 900
Phoenix, Ariz. 85004
(602) 241-2030

Field Offices:
Alameda, Calif.
Boulder City, Nev.
Phoenix, Ariz.
Reno, Nev.
San Bernadino, Calif.
Tucson, Ariz.

Resource 9:

National Cancer Institute
Call toll-free 1-800-4-CANCER

Since the National Cancer Institute set up its toll-free line, more than 1 million callers have had their questions answered or have been referred to a regional office in their area. Only four of the 21 Cancer Information Service offices cannot be reached by the toll-free number; they are:

Washington, D.C. and suburbs in Va. and Md.	636-5700
New York City	794-7982
Alaska	1-800-638-6070
Oahu, Hawaii	524-1234

The National Cancer Institute also supports research at some 60 clinics and cancer centers around the nation. For the cancer center in your area, write to the Cancer Centers Branch, Division of Resources, Centers and Community Activities, NCI, Blair Building, Room 714, Silver Spring, Md. 20205. Or phone (301) 427-8663.

Resource 10:

Environmental Protection Agency
Regional Offices

REGION I Conn., Maine, Mass., N.H., R.I., Vt.

Environmental Protection Agency
John F. Kennedy Federal Bldg., Room 2203
Boston, Mass. 02203
(617) 223-7210

REGION II N.J., N.Y., Puerto Rico, Virgin Islands

Environmental Protection Agency
26 Federal Plaza, Room 900
New York, N.Y. 10007
(212) 264-2525

REGION III Del., D.C., Md., Pa., Va., W.Va.

Environmental Protection Agency
Curtis Bldg.
Sixth and Walnut Sts.
Philadelphia, Pa. 19106
(215) 597-9800

REGION IV Ala., Fla., Ga., Ky., Miss., N.C., S.C., Tenn.

Environmental Protection Agency
345 Courtland St. N.E.
Atlanta, Ga. 30308
(404) 881-4727

REGION V Ill., Ind., Mich., Minn., Ohio, Wis.

Environmental Protection Agency
230 South Dearborn St.
Chicago, Ill. 60604
(312) 353-2000

REGION VI Ark., La., N.M., Okla., Texas

Environmental Protection Agency
First International Bldg.
1201 Elm St.
Dallas, Texas 75270
(214) 767-2600

REGION VII Iowa, Kan., Mo., Neb.

Environmental Protection Agency
324 E. 11th St.
Kansas City, Mo. 64106
(816) 374-5493

REGION VIII Colo., Mont., N.D., S.D., Utah, Wyo.

Environmental Protection Agency
1860 Lincoln St.
Denver, Colo. 80295
(303) 837-3895

REGION IX Ariz., Calif., Hawaii, Nev., American Samoa, Trust Territories of the Pacific, Guam, Northern Marianas

Environmental Protection Agency
215 Fremont St.
San Francisco, Calif. 94105
(415) 974-8153

REGION X Alaska, Idaho, Ore., Wash.

Environmental Protection Agency
1200 Sixth Ave.
Seattle, Wash. 98101
(206) 442-5810

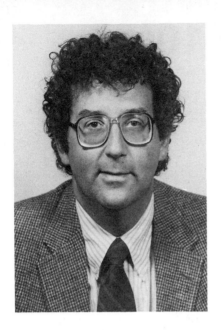

DR. PHILLIP L. POLAKOFF has long been actively involved with occupational health issues. Shortly after earning his M.D from Wayne State University, he joined the U.S. Public Health Service and became a medical investigator with the National Institute for Occupational Safety and Health (NIOSH). He later received an M.P.H. in Epidemiology from the University of California at Berkeley. He worked as an occupational physician with the Berkeley Industrial Medical Group and founded and directed the Western Institute for Occupational/Environmental Sciences, Inc. of Berkeley. Currently, Dr. Polakoff is assistant clinical professor at the Stanford University School of Medicine and the University of California at Irvine, School of Medicine. He also has a private practice in family and occupational medicine. His weekly column, Work and Health, is syndicated nationally by Press Associates, Inc. of Washington, D.C. Dr. Polakoff has published, lectured and testified extensively on job health matters.